PRAISE FOR AN E\

'Jim Dornan is as well known as ⌐
as a master obstetrician and gynae
together, add a fascinating career a   ⌐ɔɔɪ, and
what you get are tales of the unexpected, told with humour and
wisdom, around the joys and headaches that women go through in
their reproductive lives.'

Marcus Setchell, CVO, Consultant Obstetrician and Gynaecologist,
Surgeon-Gynaecologist to HM The Queen, 1990–2014

'An extraordinary selection of poignant stories collected over forty
years of frontline experience by a man whose admiration and
empathy for women, and their ability to cope with life, love and
loss during pregnancy and childbirth, shines through. The complex
medical and human dilemmas in these moving stories are explained
with warmth and humour, making them easily understandable and
accessible. You will be inspired by this book.'

Professor Lesley Regan, author of *Your Pregnancy Week by Week*

'This is the honest and engaging account of the life's work of a kind,
thinking and skilled obstetrician. Jim Dornan is a doctor who has
given so much to women and their families, whilst in return,
he has taken time – as all of us engaged in childbirth
must – to learn much from them.'

Dame Lorna Muirhead, past President of the Royal College of Midwives

'This is a beautiful book – heartwarming, heartbreaking and bursting
with humanity and tenderness. The women in this book are real
women like you or me but their stories inspire us and remind us
that, however universal or fundamental, the birth of a baby is
extraordinary. Wit, wisdom and a great deal of compassion allied
with years of obstetric practice have allowed us this wonderful
perspective on childbirth today.'

Dr Rhona Mahony, Master of the National Maternity Hospital, Dublin

'Jim Dornan's working life has been dedicated to ensuring that the
arrival of a new baby is the joy it should be, and his commitment
as one of our country's leading obstetricians has been to avoid the
tragedy of maternal death once so commonplace. His real-life stories
from the delivery room frontline are moving and inspiring, and
show just what a gift each healthy baby – and mum – is.'

Sarah Brown

Professor Jim Dornan is one of the UK's most respected gynaecologists and obstetricians. He has over forty years of experience in his field and was Director of Fetal Medicine at the Royal Maternity Hospital in Belfast for twenty years. He holds chairs at both Queen's University Belfast and the University of Ulster, is a past Senior Vice President of The Royal College of Obstetricians and Gynaecologists and continues to be active in the field of international women's health. Jim lives and continues to practise medicine in his hometown of Belfast, and is President of TinyLife, the premature baby charity for Northern Ireland, which he helped to found in 1988.

PROFESSOR **JIM DORNAN**

An Everyday
MIRACLE

Blackstaff Press

Belfast

All the events described in this book are based on my experiences.
In some cases, I have changed patients' names to safeguard
their privacy.

First published in 2013 by Blackstaff Press
4D Weavers Court
Linfield Road
Belfast BT12 5GH

With the assistance of
The Arts Council of Northern Ireland

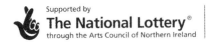

© James Dornan, 2013

James Dornan has asserted his right under the Copyright,
Designs and Patents Act 1988 to be identified as
the author of this work.

Typeset by CJWT Solutions, St Helens, England
Printed in Berwick-upon-Tweed by Martins the Printers

A CIP catalogue for this book is available from the British Library

ISBN 978 0 85640 909 7

www.blackstaffpress.com

The author is donating a percentage of his royalties to
TinyLife, the premature baby charity for Northern Ireland;
Making It Happen (Improving Maternal and Newborn Health);
and NI Leukaemia Research Fund.

This book is dedicated to women and to all that they
have achieved in the face of adversity.

Contents

Acknowledgements

In 2002 I married the amazing and beautiful Samina who hails from Asia. She is an obstetrician and gynaecologist like me, and her support for women's rights, and indeed the rights of all on a global scale, is an inspiration to me both personally and professionally.

In 2004 I was elected Senior Vice President of the Royal College of Obstetricians and Gynaecologists in London, with particular responsibility for developing global health initiatives. I shared offices with fellow officers Shaughn O'Brien and Ric Warren and those years, during which I enjoyed the benefit of their intellectual nous, friendship, wit and support, were by far the most educationally stimulating of my life.

Around the same time I met the indefatigable Nynke van den Broek from the Liverpool School of Tropical Medicine. She has been an ongoing inspiration to me and she sees no barriers to what must be done for the mothers of the world. She has led me to the conclusion that women worldwide need empowerment, education and respect far beyond that which men have given them access to thus far.

Throughout my life I have been enormously blessed. I spent my early years in an environment where caring for people was part and parcel of everyday life. My father Jim, although a highly qualified accountant, was for over thirty years General Manager of the Incorporated Cripples Institutes (now the

Northern Ireland Institute for the Disabled). My mother Clare also worked on that campus as the first occupational health carer in Northern Ireland. My parents motivated and encouraged me and their work gave me the opportunity to form many great friendships.

Whatever I have achieved, I could not have done so without many empathetic teachers at Bangor Grammar School; Alan Abraham and John Teasey stand out as truly encouraging and supportive. At Queen's University and throughout my career, Harith Lamki carefully and continually mentored me and Buster Holland and Ken Houston consistently drove me forward with encouragement, wisdom and the benefit of their experience. Rory Casement had a huge respect for all fellow human beings and women in particular and many of our coffee breaks were spent sorting out the outside world, to our satisfaction at least. These friends and colleagues taught me so much and were an ongoing inspiration to me as we worked together in the labour suites of Northern Ireland.

I met my wonderful first wife Lorna in 1970. We were blessed with many happy times together and she was an enormous support to me for many years. Her early death from cancer devastated me and our three children, Liesa, Jessica and Jamie. I think she would be immensely proud of them and what they have achieved.

This book is my first attempt at non-clinical writing and was stimulated by Alice O'Rawe from Queen's Alumni office who suggested the idea, encouraged me to put pen to paper and persuaded Patsy Horton of Blackstaff to give me a chance to publish. It has been a real pleasure to work with the whole team at Blackstaff – in spite of the liberal use of red pen!

Preface

For the last forty years I have worked as a gynaecologist and obstetrician. I feel privileged to have cared for many thousands of women, and to have personally delivered more than six thousand babies. I have treated women of all ages, from many different backgrounds and cultures, and have often been allowed a great personal insight into their lives. During my career, I have been humbled to see women struggle against adversity; I have been amazed by the strength of character that women have shown in difficult, painful, and sometimes life-threatening situations; I have shared in the heartbreak of women when they suffered tragedy and loss; and I have been part of the immense joy that women experience when they become pregnant and give birth.

If a miracle is 'an extraordinary event in the physical world that surpasses all known human or natural power', then I have observed miracles on a daily basis. As medics and midwives, we know much about how the human body works – and sometimes doesn't – but there is still much that we don't understand. Why does conception not always, or not even often, occur when we want it to do so? Why do so many women miscarry when logically they should not? Why do perfectly healthy babies all over the world occasionally, and too frequently, suddenly die in the womb when they are practically full term? Why do some placentas (afterbirths), often without any warning, become detached from the mother's womb, causing the death of the baby and putting the mother's life in grave danger? If we don't understand why these events occur, then the corollary is also true. Why do they mostly not occur? Thus, much of pregnancy and birth is indeed a miracle.

My journey to becoming an obstetrician and gynaecologist started in the early 1970s, when I began my specialist training. I was awestruck when I first saw a baby being born in early 1973. Soon after, I did a twelve-week stint as a medical student in obstetrics and gynaecology, and I knew then that this was the field that I wanted to specialise in. I have never lost the feeling that I am witnessing a miracle every time I am present or assist at a birth. I love working in an area of medicine in which the 'patient' is often healthy and happy – and excited about becoming a mother. I also love the fact that when there are problems and things go wrong, often I can do something about it. If a problem is suspected at eight o'clock in the morning, it is invariably sorted out by eight o'clock that night. Surgery has that same attraction, but a career in obstetrics and gynaecology not only includes a fair amount of surgery, it also contains strong elements of general medicine, paediatrics and psychology, and much of the research in the field is clinically based, that is focused on direct observation of the patient. Right from the start, I had the feeling that obstetrics and gynaecology could keep me fascinated for a very long time.

When my houseman year drew to a close and I became fully registered with the General Medical Council, I obtained my first six-month post as a senior house officer in obstetrics and gynaecology at Belfast City Hospital. I had many many more six- and twelve-month posts before I reached the dizzy heights of being a consultant. All in, it took six years to qualify in medicine and I worked for another twelve as a junior doctor before I became a consultant. The training programme for doctors was innovative and extremely successful in Northern Ireland. The postgraduate committee required that junior doctors applied annually for reappointment, ensuring that doctors circulated through all types of hospital and therefore experienced all types of mothers, midwives and consultants. This process allowed trainees to reconnect with the larger central teaching units on a regular basis, and also meant that trainees provided cross-fertilisation of techniques and processes between the various units.

In my forties, in common with many obstetricians, I became increasingly interested in gynaecology and in helping women to lead more comfortable physical and mental lives. Obstetrics is, in many ways, better suited to younger doctors. Long hours spent observing and dealing with long labours and effecting often strenuous interventions to deliver babies was, and is, tiring work. In a way, I grew older with my patients. Having delivered their babies, I progressed to treating them as they coped with the occasional gynaecological problems that arose after their childbearing days were over. To see women through the various stages of their lives seemed a natural progression in the provision of holistic care to them, as we moved through life together.

In 2004 I became Senior Vice President of the Royal College of Obstetricians and Gynaecologists (RCOG) in London. I took a special interest in international women's health and, as I studied the data coming in from groups such as the World Health Organisation, I became painfully aware of the crippling hardship that many women across the globe endure every day. Quite simply, an appalling number of women in the world become pregnant against their will, and practically face a death sentence when that happens. Most women in the world do not deliver in birthing units and do not have experienced personnel available to help them. Even when the personnel are available, they do not always have the necessary skills and very simple remedies that will enable them to save lives. To try to address this, I worked with the RCOG and with the Liverpool School of Tropical Medicine (LSTM) and Professor Nynke van den Broek, to develop a three- to four-day Life-saving Skills Course for international nurses, midwives and medics. The course allows faculties of obstetricians, midwives and anaesthetists from the UK and Ireland to provide hands-on, *in situ* training to midwives, clinical officers and medical officers working in resource-poor countries. Research has now shown that this type of training significantly reduces maternal loss.

Caring for women has been my life's work but I am often reminded when I talk to friends and acquaintances – both medical and non medical – how little the rest of the world knows about what actually goes on in our delivery units on a daily basis.

I hope the book gives a real sense of what it's like to work in a busy maternity unit: thinking on your feet in an emergency; helping parents to cope with the tragedy of stillbirth; sharing the joy of parents and colleagues when a healthy baby is delivered; and the comedy and laughter that comes out in the most stressful, chaotic and sometimes bizarre circumstances. Over the years, I worked with some great characters who told me terrific stories about their working lives. I've included some of those stories here, alongside my own – they capture the spirit of a different, some would say better, time.

I hope also that these stories and opinions give readers an insight into women's lives and experiences as well as a sense of some of the ongoing debates within gynaecology and obstetrics. Over the last forty years, Caesarean sections, pain relief, fetal viability and teenage pregnancy are just some of the areas in which attitudes have changed drastically, and such subjects continue to provoke much discussion both inside and outside the profession. Above all, this book is my tribute to the many women that I have cared for over the years. I hope it will give people, especially men, a greater understanding of the challenges that women face and how they cope with them, and of what needs to be done to ensure that they receive the standard of care and respect that they deserve.

A life-changing twenty-four hours

Sometimes, insights come at the most unexpected times. It was during a dinner party at a friend's house in 1990 that something happened that gave me a profound insight into how women feel about their first labour experience. Our friend Tom's mother, Anne, had died some months before, and there was a certain amount of reminiscing about her life on this particular night. Tom was an only child, something he told us he regretted to an extent. He mentioned that his mother had been very assiduous and kept little Letts diaries all her life. He had not had time to go through them yet, but the diaries were all catalogued and neatly set in rows in a wooden box in the attic.

The obstetrician in me couldn't resist asking Tom what his birth date was. It was 16 July 1942. Everyone around the table agreed that it would be fascinating if he would be willing to share his mother's diaries from that time. I couldn't help wanting to work out the likely dates of Tom's conception. You can do this using Naegele's rule. Normally the rule is used to calculate a woman's expected due date: you take the date of the first day of the woman's last period, add on a year, subtract three months and then add on seven days. However, you can also use this method to work back from the date of birth to determine the date of the first day of the last period before pregnancy. From there, you can pretty much count on the fact that conception has occurred fourteen days later. I worked out that the first day of Anne's last period, prior to the birth of Tom, must have been around late September 1941. Tom passed me the diaries and I started to leaf back to that month.

Tom, meanwhile, told us all a bit about his youth. His father had been in the army, doing his bit for King and country in South Africa. He had been in the Pioneer Corps and had been injured in a land mine incident while training in the country. His mother had often told Tom that she had, at one time, decided to remain childless, and that Tom had been an accident. It is generally recognised that in the UK, for example, about 40 per cent of pregnancies are accidents. Such pregnancies aren't planned, but the children who are born are invariably accepted and loved.

As it turned out, Anne had been fastidious about keeping her diary, and had actually circled the date of the first day of her last period in the diary. It was Monday 22 September 1941. On Sunday 21 September 1941 Anne had written in her diary, 'cleaned house very thoroughly, doing bathroom and lav etc, also a large washing of frocks and blouses'. Her husband Charlie had been away for some months at a training camp in Scotland but was due to come home the following week for a few days' leave. As a gynaecologist it is clear that any women who is trying to become pregnant, or avoid becoming pregnant will know that, if her cycle is regular, her fertile time is likely therefore to be about ten to fifteen days after the first day of her period. Anne went on to write that she was 'having afternoon tea with her friend Sadie', and noted that the 'billeting officer' called in the morning. On Tuesday 23 September 1941, being a lady of leisure and 'at that time of the month', she records in her diary that she 'stayed in bed for most of the morning, then wrote to Charlie and posted the letter just after lunch. Washed two woollen frocks and a shirt and then lay in the hammock in the afternoon.'

On Saturday 27 September 1941 she received an unexpected letter from Charlie. He wrote, 'I'm in the training camp in Liverpool on Monday morning and should be home on Tuesday.' She writes 'Oh! boy!' Come Tuesday 30 September, 1941, though, her diary contribution is despondent: 'Expecting Charlie to arrive but got a fearful disappointment when the phone rang with a wire saying he had been delayed at Stranraer and would not arrive until Wednesday.' Then in large script and capitals she wrote 'FED UP'.

But the twenty-four hours pass very quickly: 'Charlie arrived at 11 o'clock. I went to meet him and hardly recognised him in his officer's uniform. Later we had tea at the Bonne Bouche and then went to the Astoria [cinema] in the evening and saw Bing Crosby in quite a good picture.' You can imagine that as I read these entries, we all became terribly involved in the story.

On Saturday 4 October 1941 Anne and Charlie had their photos taken in the centre of Belfast. And then I think the diary entry of Sunday 5 October 1941 says it all: 'Stayed in bed late and after a good roast beef dinner we spent the afternoon with the Gardiners at Clonmill. Stayed at home in the evening and lit a fire in the drawing room. Charlie wrote several letters.' The ambience was perfect and it was the thirteenth day of Anne's cycle.

Charlie's stay was a short one. By Tuesday 7 October 1941, just forty-eight hours later, Anne recorded in her diary, 'Charlie packing, felt very lonely after he had gone.'

By this stage, there was genuine warmth developing around the table for Tom's parents. The Chinese regard their age as starting at conception so that when you are born, you are nine months old. That evening, we started to get a real understanding of that way of thinking as we read the story of Tom's beginnings.

However, by Thursday 16 October 1941, Anne still suspects nothing – 'Left a stocking in to be mended, also left short fur coat and silk skirt in with Miss Smith to be altered' – but by Saturday 23 October she is 'very anxious because something has never appeared!' Next day, she records: 'In a cold sweat about granny. Afraid am caught this time.' Tom was able to tell us that Charlie and Anne had been married for eight years at the time, so Anne had done a pretty good job in avoiding getting 'caught' until now.

Anne was by this time thirty-eight years old and it seemed pretty obvious to us all that it wasn't in her plans to have a family. Just a few days later she wrote, 'Feeling rotten, have decided to go and see Ian on Thursday.' At that time there were only a few gynaecologists in Belfast and they were all famous in their own way. Ian McClure must have been the one that Anne was attending. On Thursday 30 October Anne writes in her diary: 'Went to Ian. He gave me an examination, he is nearly sure I am pregnant, so now I will have to face it.'

All faces in the room turned to Tom who was definitely beginning to feel the reality of what his mother had always told him – that he wasn't exactly planned.

By Friday 12 December 1941 Anne was three months or fourteen weeks pregnant. She would have had a great lift by then, since any morning sickness would have been over and she would have been beginning to feel better, at least physically. I told the assembled friends that I remembered a psychiatrist telling me that women are potentially at their happiest in the middle three months of pregnancy. In fact they can be so happy that they are happier then than at any other time of their lives, and happier than a man can ever be! This is probably hormone-related but something of this feeling must also come from the relief of being out of the first three months when they are often exhausted, not yet showing, and therefore much is still expected of them, and before the final three months when they often experience some increasing discomfort. All four mothers at the table concurred heartily.

Anne wrote on Friday 12 December: 'Saw Ian, confirmed my condition, gave me a note to get extra eggs and coupons. Also to call and book a room at Johnson House on the 30 June.' Johnson House was the private wing of the Royal Maternity Hospital in

Belfast. Anne was now well into her pregnancy, and on New Year's Eve she was coping with the situation very well indeed. Charlie was still away at war: 'Bought marvellous medical book for four and nine pence at Woolworths. Had a Christmas card from Charlie, a bit late but very nice.'

By March 1942, Anne is well into the swing of the pregnancy. On Wednesday 25 March she writes, 'Bea [her close friend] came over by herself and we spent the afternoon together. Showed her the baby's trousseau.' On 31 March, though, Anne isn't feeling so well: 'Had a terrible night with my back and side, had to take three Aspirins and stayed in bed most of the morning.' The next day she went to see Ian and wrote, 'I am to leave a sample in next Wednesday.' I suspected that she had a kidney (urinary tract) infection. I was a little bemused therefore at the fact that she didn't have to leave a sample in until the following week! But the lack of urgency, I think, must have been down to the fact that antibiotics hadn't been invented, so there wouldn't have been any effective way to treat this kind of infection. Not to worry as Anne put it all down to, 'Still feeling a bit stiff, side and back, still having tinges of rheumatism.'

By the time we get to early June, at thirty-six weeks gestation, Anne is making serious preparations for the baby's arrival: 'Saw an ad for a pram and found the address. We all went to a house on the Holywood Road and saw a lovely pram, went back in the evening and I bought it for seventeen pounds.' It must have been a majestic pram to have been worth that much in 1942.

Anne was now nearing term and it was her hope that her sister, Dorrie, would stay with her during her labour. With Charlie almost on the other side of the world, and Anne being what we would term now as 'an elderly primigravida' (woman who is pregnant for the first time), she needed all the support she could get as she was beginning to feel the strain: 'Mother and I went to Ian, he doesn't need to see me again before the confinement. Letter from Dorrie to say she has strained varicose veins in her legs and won't be able to come for the event. She says to try and get Betty over [her other sister] from England. Just my luck this *would* happen.'

It seems that the pregnancy itself went very well from a physical point of view, but everyone in the room could sense that Anne was feeling a bit sorry for herself, and why shouldn't she? At least with Tom sitting there at the end of the table we knew that there would be a happy outcome eventually, at least for Tom.

On Thursday 25 June 1942, Anne records, 'I thought I seemed lower in the front this morning.' There is no doubt that women, not unnaturally, are intrigued by the birth process, and while labour itself is a bit like the proverbial piece of string and can last anything from one hour to thirty hours, the preparations for birth by the body – and the womb and pelvis in particular – go on for many weeks in the latter stages of pregnancy. Many women do 'drop' and are aware of this happening. Not that long ago, I met a woman at an antenatal clinic who asked me if I thought her baby's head had dropped. When I examined her abdominally, it was apparent that the baby's head was quite well engaged into her pelvis. She looked at me and said, 'Do you know when that happened?' I didn't answer her, as I wasn't expecting her to pick a particular moment in time. She looked at me and said, 'It happened on Wednesday night when I was in the bar at the Ivanhoe. Just after my second vodka, the head dropped! Just like that!' One of my golden rules is never to disagree with a patient, unless the situation is life-threatening, so I nodded wisely and said, 'Well indeed it has.' I left the alcohol issue for another day.

On Monday 29 June, the day before her due date, Anne writes, 'Had a letter from Charlie posted from onboard ship. Felt very weepy as it made me realise how long it would be before I see my darling again. Wrote him an aerograph and a postcard. Felt very draggy tonight.' Labour still hadn't started. However, by Wednesday 15 July, after a meal of boiled haddock and egg sauce with mushrooms, followed by blackcurrant pie, she writes in the diary, 'Had the show at 12.30 last night. Spent a very fretful night with occasional pain. Got up and dressed at 6 o'clock. Cleared the bed and made up a laundry. Made some breakfast for mother and myself at 8 o'clock. Ordered a taxi at 9.45, spent the morning at Johnson House sitting and reading on the veranda. Ian gave me a brief examination at about 12 o'clock. Real pain started at 9.30.'

The next day, Thursday 16 July, a full twenty-four hours later, Anne writes in small and neat handwriting, as it had obviously been her aim to fill the page with a very important entry: 'Spent the most ghastly night of my life. The bag apparatus ran out of gas twice at the height of my pains. Baby was born at 12.15 in the morning [Thursday 16 July]. Ian told Dorrie I had a rough time and so had he. It was far worse than my worst expectations. Was moved into a cubicle at about 6 o'clock.' Anne's mother came to visit her that evening and a cable was sent to Charlie to let him know that the baby had arrived. Tom was 9lb 12oz at birth, which might explain why both Anne and Ian experienced such a 'rough time'.

On Friday 17 July Anne writes, 'The pain in my behind this morning is awful. Not much appetite. Very uncomfortable, didn't see the baby all day.' Around the dinner table we were all relieved that Tom had been born, but we were feeling great empathy for Anne. She had delivered after the 'most horrific day of [her] life' and the pain was 'worse than her worst expectation'. She did not have her loved ones around her and she was obviously exhausted. Tom was being referred to as 'the baby'. When was all the bonding process going to occur, if ever? We didn't have to wait too long.

By Saturday 18 July Anne writes, 'Feeling a bit better today. Still having some ghastly pains at times with my stitches. Wee Tom is starting to feed well already. [The four women around the table were in tears.] I hope all will be well with him.' By Monday 22 July everyone was in tears, including me. 'Tom looks sweeter every day, I love him so.'

By Saturday 1 August 1942, Anne had been in hospital for ten days. She received a cable from Charlie saying that he had arrived in Durban. She writes in her diary, 'Sister Radcliffe came in at 6 a.m. and informed me that I was to go home tomorrow. This is a blow as I feel so weak.' There is nothing written in the diary for the next while. But all became clear on Thursday 17 September when she writes, 'Diary found, feeling my old self again, baby nine weeks old today.'

At the end of the story we all felt almost as exhausted as Anne, both physically and emotionally. It was a cathartic experience for us to read that diary, and Tom was good to allow us to do so.

In my working life I have seen nature at its most beautiful and best, and I have seen it at its roughest and toughest. The events that occur during the labour process often have a profound impact on a woman and her partner for years, if not for ever. Before epidurals became an option for women in the developed world, many women who had a great fear of childbirth sought out doctors who would provide so much sedation that there would be no bad memories to endure. I remember hearing of a senior colleague whose wife was supposedly so traumatised during labour that she chose never to have any more children – and this of course was in the days when there was not reliable contraception. The way that thousands of couples dealt with that situation was to stop having sex entirely. The colleague in question vowed that if any woman came to him asking for 'twilight sleep' during childbirth, he would willingly provide it, on the basis that while the woman might miss out on a wonderful natural birthing experience, she wouldn't have a bad one, and would at least give consideration to having more children.

Anne certainly had made her decision that Tom was to be an only child. On Thursday 4 January she wrote in her diary, 'Sold pram to Pamela for ten pounds and ten shillings.' Tom's christening card shows that he was christened on Sunday 27 December at St Columba's Parish Church, Kings Road, Knock. Reverend Alexander christened him Thomas William Oliphant. Present were Anne's mother, Auntie Dorrie, Auntie

Betty, Uncle George and Mrs Bea Harris. A note was made that 'Daddy was away in Africa'.

But while Charlie might have been physically absent in those early days, he was very much with his wife in spirit. He wrote a song for Anne while he was lying in the military hospital in North Africa in 1944 and the words speak of his longing to be home: 'From the very hour I left dear, I have been dreaming night and day, longing for that great reunion, when I come home to stay.' And he did, eventually.

In my recent working life I have used Anne's diaries as a way into talking about antenatal care and labour. The early part of her pregnancy was a time of great fear and anxiety. The middle part of her pregnancy was enjoyable and exciting. Her labour was horrific, but the outcome, for Tom at any rate, was just wonderful. Anne's unique diaries perfectly illustrate that while pregnancies and births rarely run entirely smoothly, the end result is often a happy one.

The art of obstetrics

It is a privilege to see a woman give birth and I have never forgotten my first experience of this. For me and for many in my profession, we still feel a sense that we are witnessing a miracle when we are present or assist at a birth. The majority of women in the resourced world give birth accompanied by midwives or medics. In poorly resourced parts of the world, however, most women give birth alone. Birthing attendants with proper training are hard to find, and fully equipped birthing units even harder. Europe has 15 per cent of the world's disease and 18 per cent of the total health workforce, giving us 19 healthcare practitioners per 1,000 of the population. Africa has 25 per cent of world's disease, 3 per cent of the health workforce and thus only 2.3 workers for each 1,000 of the population. It has been estimated that across thirty-six African countries there is a need for an additional one million doctors, midwives and nurses.

For varying reasons, not all women can give birth easily unaided, and midwives and obstetricians often have to use skills that have been handed down over the centuries in order to effect a safe birth. These skills, when applied in a sensitive, appropriate and efficient manner, are known as 'The Art of Obstetrics or Midwifery'.

During much of the middle part of the twentieth century, the majority of births in Ireland and the UK that occurred in domestic surroundings were attended by a midwife with the occasional timely intervention of the family General Practitioner. This trend for home confinement, for many good and some not-so-good reasons, changed during the 1960s and 1970s. Getting women to come to a birthing unit instead of delivering at home allowed them easily to access skilled help when it was needed, and hence fewer mothers and their newborns came to grief. The downside was that mothers had to leave the familiarity of the home and mobilise the family network to care for the rest of their children while they were in hospital. It would be difficult now to fully reverse this trend of hospital delivery as the majority of GPs no longer have the desire, or indeed the skills, necessary to perform a home delivery. In the 1970s, however, the vast majority of GPs in Belfast had the skills to deliver babies and used them to good effect.

In 1975, during one of my senior house officer years, I had the opportunity to do a two-week locum for a GP on the Ormeau Road in south Belfast. Teddy was a completely dedicated doctor who tended to his 'flock' and gave them the care they required and desired. He had about four thousand patients on his books and, when I went to see him before starting my locum period, he assured me that his patients were very unlikely to trouble me at night. He was right – I only got one phone call after 10 p.m. during the whole fourteen days that I was on call, and that was quite appropriate: a young child was having a severe asthma attack. Even then, the parents were embarrassingly apologetic for having bothered me.

Teddy lived above the surgery in a large three-storey detached house. His patients were of all ages and stations but, to a man, woman and child, were polite, grateful, non-threatening and mostly had genuine problems that required attention. Almost all the patients under the age of twenty-five had been delivered by Teddy, or one of his midwives, in their own homes and certainly seemed none the worse for it.

Although the locum post lasted only two weeks, I learned an awful lot about how to get the best out of the very symbiotic relationship between doctor and patient. I learnt that the best relationships were based on mutual trust. Teddy's patients trusted him to do his best, and he trusted them to be genuine and not to abuse the service. At the start of the week Teddy showed me round his surgery, gave me a quick explanation on how to deal with impacted ear wax and other minor ailments, and then pulled out his leather carpet bag from under the examination couch and said to me, 'You know what this is, don't you?' I said I didn't and he said, 'This is my obstetric kit, which I take with me when I go to do deliveries.' He knew I had started a career in obstetrics, so he gave me a look. There was a mask for giving chloroform for home anaesthesia, buccal Pitocin for inducing contractions, Heminevrin for the fits that could occur when the blood pressure was too high, suture materials and a pair of Barnes Neville forceps. He took the forceps from the bag, looked at me and said, 'You know, there is an art to obstetrics.' I nodded in agreement.

The use of forceps to help to deliver the baby and the skills to perform that manoeuvre well are a major component of the art of obstetrics. As with all arts, it is not just the manner in which one uses the instruments to effect the delivery that matters, but making sure that you are using the right instrument on the right patient, at the right time, at the right place, and in the correct manner, or deciding whether to use them at all. Forceps have been around for a few hundred years and haven't changed a lot. But then, neither have mothers and their babies or their requirements.

Sadly, the truth is that millions of women throughout the world simply die when they are unable to deliver their babies. The baby dies during the labour and then it becomes infected, and this is followed by the mother becoming infected and then she dies with the baby undelivered. Before the use of forceps, this was an even bigger problem. So when forceps were initially designed the people that used them very quickly obtained celebrity status. Their skills were much sought after and the purveyors were almost seen as magicians. The Chamberlen brothers, for example, who invented obstetric forceps, did all their forceps deliveries under a huge, black cloak, in much the same manner as photographers taking photographs, so that the secret of their use could not be shared with other doctors or observers. They went on to have a monopoly in the art of forceps use for three generations.

Just as there have been no major design changes in women, so there have been few design changes in forceps. The vast majority of forceps have two curves: one curve to go around the baby's head and another curve to take into account the delivery of the baby through the natural curve of the mother's pelvis and birth canal. Fenestrae, or windows, were put in to allow space for the baby's ears, and the forceps blades are inserted one at a time. When they are placed on the baby's head, in the correct manner, in the right place, at the ideal angle, they naturally lock together. This is a key point in their use.

Even the word forceps can engender horror and fear in women but probably 10 per cent of the population of the western world has been delivered with their use, and the vast majority of both babies and mothers are left with no permanent damage. Used properly in skilful hands, forceps are life-savers. Much of the skill in their use comes from their correct application, taking into account the position of the fetal head and whether any asynclitism needs to be allowed for. Asynclitism refers to the position of the baby's head, when it is leaning over to one side more than another. Once the forceps are applied and locked, the actual delivery of the baby's head is mostly down to simply adding to the maternal effort, and pulling in the correct direction. These skills are somewhat different to those required to effect delivery with the ventouse vacuum device. In simple terms the ventouse is used like a sink plunger that is applied to the back of the baby's head. The skill with using forceps is mostly in the application of the instrument, with the delivery being almost a process of extracting the forceps with the baby following along. Whereas, with the ventouse, although skill is required to apply the vacuum cup, it is in guiding the baby through the birth canal that most skill is required. I have intentionally gone into some detail here so that the reader can appreciate the next part of the story.

I told Teddy that I hoped that I was going to spend the next decades of my life perfecting the art of obstetrics. He assured me that it wouldn't take that long to teach me! He then went on to tell me how the forceps worked. Teddy told me that difficult labours invariably seem to occur in the middle of the night – I think he was right there, and it is a lonely time for all involved. He continued, 'You get a phone call from the midwife to tell you that your patient has been pushing like a Trojan for maybe a couple of hours and is just exhausted and needs help. You get out of bed, get dressed, pop into the surgery, collect the obstetric bag and drive to the mother's house. Usually the man of the house is standing at the door to let you in, and you go upstairs to the main bedroom where the midwife and the mother are equally exhausted. You examine the mother, and often find that the baby's head is stuck, and despite the apparent adequacy of the mother's passage, and the desire of the baby to be delivered, you find that the mother's uterine contractions are on the wane and at that least another 20 per cent of effort is required all round.'

Teddy then lifted the forceps and demonstrated in detail how to apply them. 'You take one of the Barnes Neville forceps blades in your left hand and slip it in alongside the baby's ear, usually its left ear on the left side of the mother's pelvis first, for reasons that are a little bit technical to tell you about since you're only starting. Then you take the second forceps blade and slip it in down the other side of the baby's head.'

Now even at that stage of my career, I knew that the blades should – indeed must – lock together before any attempt is made to deliver the head. In fact, the act of the forceps locking implies that they are highly likely to have been applied correctly. But Teddy looked at me in a scholarly manner and said, 'Having applied both the blades, sometimes they don't lock, and that's when the art of obstetrics comes in – getting the baby's head out with the blades apart!' It was an astute comment in many ways – I'm sure that in the middle of the night a certain modification of 'the art' was required to deliver the baby's head in this way on occasions. In a hospital setting, however, if the forceps didn't lock you would readdress the position of the baby's head and then review how to progress with that particular delivery.

So Teddy was right in one way – it would indeed require quite an art to deliver the baby's head with the blades apart! Much in medicine in general and obstetrics in particular is put down to '*secundum artem*'. In other words, one often develops the art as it is required. Teddy was obviously a master of the process. In the two weeks I worked for him, I only heard praise from his patients for his ability, dedication, caring and indeed for his application of the 'art of obstetrics' – only one of the many, many arts he surely possessed.

Fame on the Falls Road

In the 1960s, when I was doing my medical training, students were not introduced to real patients until near the end of their third year of study. Up until that time, typically, the medical undergraduate course was quite cold and heavily academic. The only real bodies we saw were the ones kindly donated for medical research that we dissected as the main part of our anatomy programme.

I remember well the first time I walked into the dissecting room. It was extremely cold and incredibly quiet, and I don't think I actually looked at my assigned body for the first hour. Rather, I stared at the floor or my textbook until I eventually summoned up some courage and ventured a peek. It wasn't the very first cadaver I had been close to but its appearance was a shock to me – only then did I get a real sense of how skilled funeral parlour morticians are at presenting a corpse.

It was, therefore, with a mixture of trepidation and excitement that we ventured onto the wards of the hospital for the first time during our third year. I took to it straight away – the warmth and the general buzz and bustle instantly made the wards a place that I wanted to be. I rapidly realised that medics and hospital staff regularly used humour to break the spell of gloom and despondence that is often present in grave situations. It's how the human spirit deals with the raft of ever-changing emotions as patients get worse and better at frequent intervals and rates.

Prior to entering the wards for the first time, I don't think I had ever considered that humour was a necessary and frequent element in the complex relationship between patient and doctor. That discovery delighted me completely. I am a great believer and proponent of Voltaire's observation that 'It is the physician's role to keep the patient amused while awaiting nature to effect a cure.' Following my first ward round, however, I realised that the use of humour could be a two-way street.

Patients in those days were treated in Victorian single-gender wards, and the beds always seemed to be full. There were twenty to twenty-four beds in each ward, sufficiently close together to allow intimate conversation, the sharing of cigarettes, newspapers and biscuits, and the simple spread of infection. There was also just enough room for twelve to sixteen medical students to stand around the bed during a ward round.

Throughout my working life, no matter what bed cuts or bed expansions have been implemented by hospital management, there always seems to be 'pressure on beds'.

Many ailments can now be addressed at the outpatient and community level, but at the same time there are many more surgical and interventional options available to patients. Also the home environments from which patients come, and to which they hope to return after treatment, have changed dramatically over the decades. The NHS, at its formation in 1948, was an oasis for much of the population, who had endured a lifetime of outside toilets, only cold running water, and the sharing of a bedroom, often with many siblings. Coming into hospital was certainly a harrowing experience, but it also gave patients access to a welcoming and clean environment, along with warmth, regular food, and love and encouragement from at least the nurses, if not all the medics.

Hospital also brought patients into contact with some fairly serious and well-regarded consultants and it was just such a consultant that took my colleagues and me on our first ward round in April 1969 on wards 15/16 of the old Royal Victoria Hospital corridor. These ward rounds were major occasions, consisting of a group of twenty- and twenty-one-year olds traipsing down the ward following the great man, with our brand new, clean, starched, white coats, and new shiny stethoscopes bulging out of our pockets. They confirmed my opinion of the character and personalities of my fellow students. Those who regularly sat in the front two rows during lectures, with blue padded anoraks on, were now right at the very front of the ward round, while those of us who usually sneaked into the back of lectures, clasping a third cup of coffee to get over the rigours of the night before, were now slinking in towards the back.

Consultants were in their element during these rounds. This was their arena, and they stood with their equally freshly starched white coats fully buttoned up, with one hand on the head of the bed, and the other hand free to point at random at various students to see if we could be annihilated just one more time before the coffee break. At times the patient was almost secondary to the real theatre in progress.

The consultant in question, Mr Wainwright, was taking our first ward round, and was due to operate on the irrepressible Joe Moffat the following afternoon. Joe had spent his life working at the docks. He was a thin and wiry individual, but looked as strong as an ox. He had gone through his adult life complaining of terrible heartburn and gastritis. The wonderful proton-pump inhibitors, which help to reduce gastric acid production, had not been discovered, and so Joe's stomach had been producing acid non-stop, which was irritating his stomach ulcer. He lived on handfuls of white chalk tablets of calcium carbonate that attempted to neutralise the acid, in between an excess of pints of Harp lager and Ulster fries. The only thing left to Joe, and indeed to us medical students who often suffered a similar affliction for exactly the same reasons, was the consumption of these chalk products in the form of tablets or liquid. Milk of Magnesia and Rennies were in everyone's pockets in those days.

Mr Wainright had made his name by carrying out an operation known as a Highly Selective Vagotomy, which involved cutting the nerves that supply the stomach's acid production system.

The name of the operation in itself impressed us and suggested that a major degree of skill was required to perform the procedure. We certainly understood from our surgical lectures and work in the dissecting room what exactly the surgeon was intending to do, but we hadn't seen him in action at that stage.

The surgeon spent about five minutes allowing Joe to give us a history. His lifestyle was fairly typical of its time. He smoked forty Gallaher's Blues cigarettes per day, consumed 'a few' pints of lager on a daily basis, and then indulged in some serious drinking on a Saturday night. His diet could not have been described as healthy. All in all Joe, at the age of thirty-two, was in serious need of some relief as he was having to declare himself unavailable for dock work on a fairly regular basis.

Joe had somewhere between five and seven children, which again was pretty common in those days. So it was important that Joe was patched up and returned to his family as soon as possible, so he could continue in his role as the main provider.

At the completion of the care discussion, and Mr Wainright's subsequent inquisition of us with our sparse knowledge, he asked Joe to show us a hidden condition that was rare and was to prove illuminating. As well as his gastric problems, Joe had a very large swelling in one of his testicles, which was filled with fluid. It was 'the size of a melon' we were informed – in those days, before widespread imaging techniques were available, all tumours and masses were described through comparisons to fruit and vegetables.

Mr Wainwright took two sheets of A4 and rolled them up into a tube. Joe seemed quite happy to allow the nurse, on instruction, to undo his pyjama cord and for us to see him in his – almost – full glory. By putting an eye to one end of the paper tube and placing the other end on the scrotum, and then shining a pen torch through the testicle, we were able to see the pink light shining through the hydrocele, thus confirming that it was fluid-filled. This is called transillumination, and its presence confirmed that the mass in Joe's scrotum was indeed a benign hydrocele that was simply full of fluid. In turn, all sixteen of us queued up to look through the paper tube at Joe's nether regions. Joe himself was entrusted to hold the torch at the other side so that he didn't have to have sixteen pairs of hands manipulating his scrotum any further. We were all well impressed with this clinical sign, which was clearly demonstrated. Although the skills that I obtained that day, I admit, I have never required since.

At the end of the process, Joe closed his pyjamas and pulled the sheets back up with a degree of heartfelt satisfaction. At the conclusion, Mr Wainwright turned to Joe, and in a fairly patronising manner said, 'There you are now Joe; tomorrow we will have you in theatre. We will sort that stomach problem out for you, and don't worry about a thing, while we are there we will remove that hydrocele from your scrotum.'

In response to this, an indignant Joe looked up at Mr Wainwright, and in a broad Belfast accent said, 'Well you can fix the stomach if you like, but you can keep your hands off my balls, for them's the biggest balls on the Falls Road and you're not touching them.' We all burst out laughing. Joe stood his ground, and Mr Wainwright became quite obviously flustered, which gave us a fair amount of pleasure. He just looked at Joe and said, 'I will be back to talk to you later.'

Later came and went, and Joe kept his magnificent hydrocele. I am pretty confident that the light shone on, and indeed through, Joe for many years to come on the Falls Road.

Is it a boy or a girl?

Fifty years ago, most women got married in their twenties and very quickly afterwards attempted to become mothers. Their official sexual and reproductive lives started with the words 'I do'. If, twenty-four months later, pregnancy had not occurred, and infertility treatment was not successful, adoption was often the way forward. When I started out on my career some forty years ago, in the mid-1970s, adoption still offered the best opportunity for childless couples to create a family. It was possible to try artificial insemination – a medic manually inserted the sperm of the husband or a donor into to the cervix (neck of the womb) and the woman was given drugs to stimulate the release of eggs – but the success rate was low. There was little one could offer the sub-fertile man. For a woman with apparently blocked Fallopian tubes the only hope was fairly major open surgery. It is not surprising that when a couple started out on the often-fruitless road of fertility treatment, many would also put their names on the adoption agency's list.

Mostly those children available for adoption were the result of an out-of-wedlock relationship. Back then, being an unmarried mother or the child of an unmarried mother brought with it social stigma and many single mothers – often after untold heart searching – gave up their babies for adoption, mostly to loving parents who cherished them. I have personal experience of adoption in that my younger sister was adopted by my parents and my first wife was also an adopted child. My mother miscarried in 1962 in mid-pregnancy when I was thirteen years of age. My parents were heartbroken, but I remember vividly, within a few months, being taken one evening to a local nursing home and being introduced to my new sister. I loved her instantly, as did my parents. I have known many many adopted women and men, who have had hugely positive, productive lives, and have given and received love beyond compare.

Now, however, adoption is a much less common way for childless parents to address their situation. This is due to two factors. The first is that there are there fewer children, at least in Britain and Ireland, who need to be adopted – a situation that has come about in part because of the removal of the stigma around being an unmarried mother. The second factor is the pioneering work of Patrick Steptoe and Robert Edwards who developed IVF in the 1970s – the first test-tube baby, Louise Brown, was born in 1978 – and changed the world of reproduction forever. This in turn has led to a redefinition of infertility. Many women are leaving attempts at childbearing till their late thirties and so this advice is redundant, certainly for women approaching the end of their fourth decade. Investigation can now bring hope, and bring it quickly. The resulting plethora of reproductive techniques that has followed the early work of Steptoe and Edwards has given huge hope to couples with fertility problems worldwide.

The sweeping advances in reproductive techniques over the last forty years now make it possible to create designer babies, and, outside the UK, sex selection through pre-implantation genetic diagnosis (PGD) is all the rage in many countries, and in Asia in particular, where the sex of the baby is often considered to be of vital importance. In much of the world, producing a male child is not just a matter of desire, it is something that some people are prpared to go to any lengths – not all of them legal – to achieve. PGD is now used, for better or for worse, widely throughout the world for this purpose.

When fertilisation occurs, the resultant egg quickly starts a process of mitosis, dividing into two cells, then four, then eight, sixteen, and so forth. At the eight-cell stage, one cell can be extracted in the laboratory and the genetic code, which includes the sex of the potential baby, can be deciphered. At one end of the spectrum, PGD techniques allow for the detection of lethal abnormalities and, at the other, they allow for the creation of designer babies (it is now theoretically possible to choose not just the sex of a baby but the colour of its hair and its eyes). Such developments take us into difficult ethical territory. Some thirty years ago, when much of this research was still in its infancy, such advances seemed to me Orwellian, a step too far. However, I met Enoch Powell at a dinner in Belfast and took the opportunity to ask him about the issue: 'In the next few decades it will be possible to take a sample of the mother's blood at the time of her first missed period, that is in very early pregnancy. There will already be cells from the embryo in that sample. It will be possible to extract those cells, and by DNA replication, the next day we will know everything there is to know about that child's potential medical future life. Do you think that government should bring in legislation to prevent such research?' He gave me the most incredibly sensible answer: 'One cannot prevent man's desire to find out everything there is to know around about him by using his intellect and scientific ability, which may well include getting right down to the very source of life itself. However, when, in trying to find those answers, man creates something that can, will or may, have an effect on all mankind, then government must intervene to curb it, but only then.' I was greatly taken by his answer, and I have had no reason since that time to argue with his logic.

There are some horrific consequences to the desire for a child of a particular sex in many places, solutions that can involve men depriving women of their sexual and reproductive rights. Many cultures value the birth of a son over a daughter, and in order to maximise the chances of this occurring, many women in Asia are being encouraged and sometimes forced to undergo termination of their pregnancies following the ultrasound identification of the sex of the baby in early pregnancy.

I was holding a gynaecology clinic in a rural part of the northwest of Ireland some years ago. One of the women who came to see me was a farmer's wife called Matilda. While taking her family history I asked her if she had any sisters. She replied, 'I have three in a way, but in another way I have three brothers.' I was a bit confused and asked her to expand. She went on to explain to me that her parents lived on a farm and her 'mother' had given birth to three boys before she came along. She had been very keen to have a girl, but it just didn't happen. She went on that to tell me that her mother and her 'aunt' lived on farms next to one another, and that her mother had three boys and her aunt had three girls. Serendipitously both her mother and her aunt found themselves pregnant at the same time with their fourth children. Her mother was desperate for a girl and her aunt was desperate for a boy. The two women delivered within a few days of each other but they each delivered a child of the same sex as their older children. It seems that without any fuss, each family quite simply swapped their latest additions, and so Matilda was brought up very successfully by her mother, while her aunt (her biological mother) continued to live on the adjoining farm and raised Mathew as her own. Matilda was incredibly well-balanced, and both she and her male cousin had managed to go through life without issues, counselling, behavioural problems or tantrums.

There is an increasing trend among parents to be informed of the sex of their baby before birth. Personally, I think it's a good idea. My experience is that it improves bonding and allows parents to really focus in on the baby as a person, and I only remember one woman in thirty-nine years who was genuinely and almost inconsolably disappointed when she discovered that the sex of the baby was not what she wanted. The vast majority of parents quickly adapt to what nature provides.

Some years ago, I carried out a scan on a woman in mid-pregnancy, who already had six sons at home. As you might expect, she had a very practical attitude to life, and a good no-nonsense approach to pregnancy. While scanning her, the gender of the baby was pretty apparent to me – it was fairly obvious that she was about to have a seventh son. 'Can you tell what sex the baby is doctor?' she said. I replied that I could. She said, 'Okay, you might as well tell me. What is it?' I said, 'Well actually, it's another boy. Congratulations.' She replied, 'That's great, doctor, that's okay. The boys will be delighted. One more for them to kick the ball about with.' But I wondered was she not just a wee bit disappointed, so I thought I would share out the responsibility somewhat. There wasn't much said for the next ten seconds or so, and since I don't enjoy long silences, I said, 'Of course, we must remember that it's the man who "decides" whether it's a boy or a girl. The gender choice apparatus is in the head of the sperm.' She looked at me knowingly and said, 'Aye, you're right, doctor. Sure you can only work with the materials that you're given.' What a wonderful statement, I thought then, and have often thought since. That statement covers a multitude of situations that I come across on a daily basis. In the past, so many of the problems that women had were viewed by men with an attitude of 'You better get that seen to', when in fact it should have been 'We need to get that seen to'.

Meanwhile, there has been no truer or more practical expression shared with me by any woman over the years than that by that mother of six … and counting.

The history that was too perfect

In the 1970s there were literally hundreds of nursing homes throughout Ireland in which pregnant woman could have their babies delivered, or indeed simply rest a while in preparation for birth before moving to a birthing unit nearby. One such establishment was situated about five miles outside a border town in which I worked during the late 1970s. Every sizeable town in Ireland probably had a similar facility.

In 1970s Ireland, when a young girl found herself to be pregnant outside wedlock, she had limited options. She could urgently marry the father, which many women did. Such marriages produced many so-called premature babies, born six months after the wedding day but weighing 4.5kg (9½lb)! The next most common choice for an unmarried expectant mother was to carry the baby to term, and then allow it to be put up for adoption. This difficult decision would be taken after much soul-searching and after a vast amount of advice from medical practitioners, family, friends and clergy. In the case of the family, often even the girl's mother would keep the news from her husband, and the daughter would be sent off to 'London to do a course' or something similar.

A final option was abortion. Many, many young girls and women in Ireland and the United Kingdom died from backstreet abortions until the 1967 Abortion Act was passed in

Great Britain. Whatever else the introduction of this Act did, at a stroke it halted the colossal and tragic loss of young female life from criminal abortion. The option to have an abortion was – and still is – frequently availed of by women from across the whole island of Ireland, though in almost all cases they had to, and still have to, travel to England for the procedure.

A few weeks after arriving at the local hospital where I was to work for the year, I was asked to see a young girl, Rosalind, in the casualty unit one night, as she considered herself to be in labour. Rosalind was a shy eighteen-year-old, of slight build with pale, curly blond hair. Each time I saw her, she gave the appearance of being preoccupied. She was an unmarried farmer's daughter who lived in the next county, but she was spending her antenatal period in one of the nursing homes described above.

In the weeks before I first saw her she had apparently frequently come to casualty with the symptoms, but not the signs, of labour. Her histories, social and medical, were indeed very suggestive of her baby being at full term. I was impressed that she was able to tell me accurately the date her last menstrual period had begun, the date on which she had found out she was pregnant, the date she first felt the baby move and her actual expected date of confinement, for not many mothers, particularly young ones, knew this kind of detail.

Examination of Rosalind's pregnant abdomen confirmed a good-sized baby and certainly it might have been in or around the size of a term baby. A term baby, though, could be anything from six to twelve pounds, so size alone wasn't much of a guide. The baby was presenting headfirst and its head was not engaged in Rosalind's pelvis. Again, 97 per cent of babies present headfirst and very few of them are properly engaged until the mother is established in labour so those findings didn't really help me determine exactly the gestation of this particular pregnancy.

I personally felt no contractions, apart from Rosalind herself tightening up her abdominal muscles in a regular manner in an effort to show me that the baby was on its way. Examination of the cervix showed that it was not dilating. All Rosalind's observations and investigations were normal and I reassured her that she was not in labour, even though she was convinced that this was her due date. There was no doubt that Rosalind deeply *wanted* to be in labour and was quite distressed and a bit annoyed with me for denying that she was.

Ultrasound use was in its infancy in those days and access to it in the hospital was very patchy. It took many decades before this situation was addressed, and even now, incredibly, its use is not accepted by all healthcare professionals. Midwives on the ground, for example, love using it but their political seniors had traditionally, certainly in the twentieth century, a deep distrust for any gizmo with an electric wire protruding from it. There was a strong feeling that anything electrical, and therefore de facto unnatural, was to be shunned because it formed part of the dreaded medicalisation of childbirth.

That day, however, I was able to carry out a scan on Rosalind and the baby looked to be well grown and in a healthy environment. I told Rosalind that I would visit her in her nursing home during the following week or the week after. She said that when I did she would show me her diary, which would prove that by the time of my proposed visit, she would be well past her expected date of confinement.

Seven days came and went and Rosalind made no further attempts to gain admission to the maternity unit. I went to see her the next Friday afternoon on my way back home for the weekend. On my way to visit her at the home, I took the opportunity of carrying out a few other visits following a request from one of the GPs in the district. These visits were known as 'domiciliaries' and could be ordered by the GP when they wanted a consultant to visit the home of a female patient who had a logistical problem getting to the hospital. In the rural area in question I always tried to do my allotted domiciliaries on a Friday afternoon, as those who you visited were so pleased to see you that the whole afternoon turned into a social event, and it was not unusual to be offered a glass of whisky or poteen as well as numerous cups of tea, homemade apple tart and other sweet treats.

I called to see Rosalind as planned and found her sitting up in bed. She immediately said, 'Dr Dornan, I want to show you something. As soon as I found out I was pregnant, my mother was so distraught that she sent me over to stay with relatives in London, but I became so sick and lonely that she eventually told my father and he told her to bring me home. They were still embarrassed about me being pregnant and so I have been in this home since I came back. But they are beginning to wonder why this baby isn't coming out when it should. Everything I am telling you is true, because I wrote it all down here in this diary and look – here it is.'

Rosalind opened her bedside drawer and produced a fresh-looking Letts diary for that year and every piece of information that she had given me – the date of her last period, the date of conception, the date she found out she was pregnant, the date when she told her mother, the date when she went to London, and so on – was there, recorded in her handwriting. She did, however, make two rather large and important mistakes: firstly, the only facts that were in the diary were the pregnancy ones that she had related to me – no other events had been logged. There wasn't even a 'went to church', 'went out with Mary' or 'had a good dance last night' that might have given some authenticity to the events recorded. Secondly, she had written all the entries in the same red biro, and therefore it was pretty obvious that she had written all the entries at the same time. As gently as possible, I pointed out that my observations suggested that the diary had been completed retrospectively and that all entries had been made on the same occasion. Rosalind blushed.

One thing the diary did do was to provide me with the reasons why she so desperately wanted to be delivered weeks early. Quite simply, nature had been playing tricks on her. When she missed a period or two, she assumed she was pregnant, was distraught and told her mum, who then swiftly spirited her to London. In reality, though, she was not pregnant when she went to London but was by the time she left! Hence her desire to have the baby at the time she thought, and hoped, it was due.

We chatted for a long time and I made it clear to her that it was my own view that she still had many weeks of her pregnancy to go. Understandably she was concerned because she knew this would have implications in relation to what she had told her parents about the time, place and person involved at the conception. Still, it would not have implications otherwise as the baby was still going to be offered for adoption.

Time went on and I was delighted that I was on call the evening Rosalind eventually went into labour, some six weeks later. I was in the room with her but she certainly didn't need my obstetrical expertise. She pushed mightily, as they say, and delivered a beautiful baby girl who weighed in at 9lb 12oz.

It is a matter of great sadness to me in retrospect that Rosalind had her baby when the practice was not to show the mother the baby at any stage when it was going for adoption. Amazing efforts were made to prevent young, often frightened mothers, from seeing their newborn babies. These mothers could feel the babies move inside their wombs, they could work so hard to deliver them, they could feel their warmth, they could hear them cry, they could smell them. But they couldn't see them. While the vast majority of staff working in the maternity units were hugely empathetic to these young mums giving birth, there were great efforts made to shield the mother from seeing her newborn. Sheets and drapes were held up while the baby was spirited from the delivery room. Even then it all seemed so wrong. I always thought of my sister and my wife, both of whom were adopted, and of what their birth mothers must have gone through. In Rosalind's case a green material shield was erected to prevent her getting even a glimpse of the baby. I did however describe the newborn baby in great detail to Rosalind and she appeared very calm and content. Resigned.

Exactly the same efforts were made when a baby was stillborn or was known to have a life-threatening abnormality. It wasn't really until the 1980s that attitudes to birth culture started to change, a shift in which Esther Rantzen played a key part. She and her team challenged the accepted idea that babies who were born dead should not be seen or nursed. Eventually, the new ways of managing these kinds of birth that came about by her efforts were extended to include babies who could not survive after birth because of fetal abnormalities who were going to be adopted, and indeed, at last, to babies for adoption. Adoption is rare enough nowadays in the world in which I work, but at least when it does occur, there is huge compassion and empathy openly provided for the birth mother and her family.

I saw Rosalind six weeks later for a postnatal check-up at the hospital, which was normal practice then, and I believe a valuable one, and which has now been deemed to be of little clinical benefit by the powers that be. We had a chat about the antenatal period and in fact we had a good laugh about the 'diary that wasn't'. Her parents had been just super, even after they had worked out the implications of the eleven-month pregnancy! She and her dad had become closer than ever. He was encouraging her to take up further education and she planned to go to the local technical college night classes to get more qualifications.

Society has evolved hugely since those days and while some attitudes and practices from that era now seem unnecessarily cruel, many people were doing what they thought best in the circumstances in which they found themselves. Rosalind was a star, a resourceful clever star, and a great mother who gave her daughter as good a start in life as was available and possible at that time and in that environment.

The touch of the Master's hand

Pope John Paul II came to Ireland in 1979 – a visit that is still talked about. A third of the population turned out in Phoenix Park, Dublin, to see the great man, and I am fairly sure that about half of the baby boys born in Ireland that year were christened John Paul.

During his visit, the Pope conducted a massive outdoor Mass in Drogheda, County Louth, on Saturday 29 September. While this event had many positive knock-on effects in general, it had special significance for two births in particular. I believe that a baby was delivered at the Mass itself, and in nearby Newry, where I was working at Daisy Hill Hospital, it had repercussions for one other heavily pregnant woman.

Some days before the event in Drogheda, because of the expected mayhem on the roads, the hospital took the unusual step of offering Angela McDermott a Caesarean section as the method of delivery of her second child. Angela had undergone an emergency Caesarean section for the birth of her first child because her baby had developed heart irregularities during labour. This problem in itself would definitely not have been a reason to perform a repeat Caesarean section, and in 1979 the vast majority of women who had a Caesarean section for their first birth were encouraged – closer to informed, truth be told – to try for a vaginal birth for their second baby. The concept of 'choice' had not entered our clinical vocabulary at that stage. All decisions about possible route of delivery were based totally on obstetrical indications. The prime route of delivery was accepted as the vaginal one, and a Caesarean was only contemplated when the former was considered unsafe. This provided obstetricians with a very pure approach in many ways.

The concept of choice was actually introduced by those who considered that there was too much medical interference in childbirth, and wanted women to have a greater number of natural options. However, to every action there is an equal and opposite reaction. And so, while one group of mothers have increasingly chosen to have a birth that is as natural as possible, so another group of mothers have increasingly found their voice and asserted their choice *not* to go the natural route. This latter development hasn't impressed those who favour the natural route, but they do have to be gently reminded at times that they started it!

Obstetricians and midwives are increasingly being put under pressure by management to turn the clock back to some extent, and only perform Caesareans when there are strong clinical indications. There is a well-rooted belief that Caesareans cost more, and in an increasingly cost-conscious NHS, perceived costly non-essential procedures are being questioned intensely. This all sounds very fair, but unfortunately you can often get data to say what you want. When assessing the cost of a Caesarean, often health economists include *all* Caesareans and compare their cost with monies spent on *all* vaginal births. However, an emergency Caesarean performed at the conclusion of a long and protracted labour at 3 a.m. on a Sunday morning, complicated by numerous interventions, is always going to be more expensive than an elective procedure performed at 10 a.m. on a Monday morning. At last, data from North America is coming through to support the assertion that when these considerations are factored in, there is negligible difference in cost. Hopefully this information will soon be widely understood and will lead to an honest clinical debate about the whys and wherefores of Caesareans, untarnished by arguments of cost.

The choice agenda promoted by the natural childbirth lobby sounds very correct and 'on message' in theory, but the genie of Caesareans is out of the bottle and the vast majority of women who have undergone the procedure – whether with strong, moderate, weak or no clinical indications – are extremely happy with their birth experience. Just as the majority of women who have had a natural birth are happy with their experience. It's a hard circle to square!

Forty years ago, though, we really did a lot of thinking before agreeing to repeat a Caesarean on a woman who had no pressing clinic need. Angela was one of those. In mid-September 1979 I saw Angela at the antenatal clinic. She was getting near term and, in any other circumstances at that gestation, I would have left her for another while in the hope that she would go into labour herself. I remember she said, 'Doctor, I live up in the hills. We don't even have a phone. What happens if I go into labour while the Pope's in Drogheda? They tell me there will be a million people in the field when he arrives and that's just a few miles from where I live. And my midwife says she thinks my baby's very big. You know, would it not be easier for all if I just had another Caesarean? Sure it took very little out of me last time.'

My immediate reaction, born out of my training, was, 'Well now, Angela, you're a physically well-equipped woman, and honestly there's no real reason to do a Caesarean or even induce your labour at this stage.' But she didn't give up. 'Could you not ask the consultant, Mr Holland? My mother says he's a lovely man.'

I went to see Buster (Mr Holland's nickname, given to him because of how big he was when he was delivered), expecting to give the response that, as there was no indication to do a Caesarean, Angela would have to wait, and I would have been quite happy to relay this response to her. Mothers and patients in 1979 did exactly what consultants told them. I would be off the hook.

To my surprise, however, Buster listened to the clinical facts and weighed up the social circumstances and said, 'Well, we don't want a kerfuffle when the Pope's in town, do we? You know, I have a feeling about this. Tell her to come in next week, and if she's not favourable for induction of labour, we'll do a Caesarean before the great man arrives.' I took the message back to Angela. You would have thought I had given her the Freedom of Newry.

Some days before 29 September, Angela came up to the unit, and was found not be suitable for induction. A Caesarean was planned for the next day. I remember well that the sister in labour ward and the anaesthetist were less than impressed with the decision. Sister was old-school and believed that it was not just a woman's lot to give birth naturally, but her duty, and as for the anaesthetist, well to be fair, in 1979 the operation was a bigger deal than it is now, and a full general anaesthetic was the order of the day.

On the day of the operation, Angela was unaware of the air of quiet discontent and went to sleep oblivious to the internal politics. I don't want to provoke squeamishness, but I do need to explain a little of how the operation works. Normally we incise the skin, then the fat layer, and then what is known as the sheath. The sheath protects the abdominal muscles below it. Having split this muscle down the middle we incise two thinnish layers known as the peritoneum. One layer acts as an envelope for all the bowel contents, and the other acts as an envelope for individual organs. Below this latter layer is the muscular womb, which we normally go through to find the baby surrounded by its membranes and fluid.

Having incised Angela's first layer of peritoneum I was stunned to see, staring at me through *only* the membranes, the haunting though beautiful image of Angela's baby floating in what looked like pea soup. The second layer of peritoneum and the womb muscle layers were nowhere to be seen – just the baby staring at us through the membranes. By simply touching the membranes they broke and we quickly sucked out the pea soup from in and around the baby's nose and mouth and delivered him. He cried immediately, no problems, and then we put Angela back together, again without any problems. This was, in today's parlance, a 'near miss'.

Afterwards we all streamed into the sanctuary of the rest room where we sat down and discussed the case with liberal use of the word *if*. Quite simply, the scar that Angela had from her first Caesarean section had been about to give way totally, dehisce or rupture. This can happen in rare cases but only does so after the mother has been in labour for a prolonged period. So why did it happen without labour in this case? The pea soup that we had seen around the baby in the womb was meconium (fetal bowel movement material). This is a common enough occurence after a mother passes her due date, but is pretty rare before that time. It is also potentially dangerous as meconium can be an irritant if inhaled into the baby's lungs.

So many maybes, so many what ifs. What if Angela had experienced strong contractions before we did the operation? What if she had not had a Caesarean? What if her labour had occurred in a traffic jam the next day? Realistically, Angela and the baby could have died.

After the birth, Angela and her new son continued to thrive. We didn't take her through all the ifs and maybes just then, but we did share our delight and relief at the outcome. In particular we told Angela that her choice to request a Caesarean section had been a good one, and that Buster's decision to agree to it had been a good one. We also told her that the Pope's choice to come to Drogheda on the 29 September 1979 had been a good one, and when we heard that she decided to call her son John Paul? Well, it was her choice.

Butterflies

Once a woman knows that she is pregnant, her and her partner's thoughts naturally turn to the question, 'Is my/our baby all right?' Increasingly this really means 'Is my/our baby *all* right?" It is our society's attitude to newborns not being *all* right that provides obstetricians with a complete clinical rainbow of responses to that question. Sometimes, unfortunately, the baby is not *all* right. Many pregnancies in which the baby is not all right end in miscarriage in the first months. However, up to 5 per cent of all newborn babies have some health issues.

Less than 1 per cent of all babies have a serious, even life-threatening problem that is diagnosed antenatally or at birth; the kind of problem that means huge challenges for all concerned. When this does happen, obstetricians and midwives encounter a range of reactions and responses from parents. Some are overwhelmingly positive: 'if it's God's will we will accept it'; 'we will take what comes doctor'; 'we will do everything we can for the baby, doctor' and 'we will let nature take its course'. But we also frequently hear, 'can you assure me everything is normal?'; 'what tests can we have done to make sure everything is normal doctor?'; 'I couldn't have another disabled baby, doctor'; 'I can't leave my children with the burden of caring for two disabled siblings'; 'I will only get pregnant if you guarantee me that the baby will be normal'; 'What do you mean by risk, doctor?' and

'Can you guarantee me that everything will be all right?'

My job, and that of my colleagues, is difficult in such circumstances but there are two principles by which we try to abide. First, we give parents as much information as they request about the condition that might affect their baby. No more and no less. Second, we don't impose our own personal agenda on the decision-making process unless it is vital to do so to save the mother's life. We have to be sure that we make the parents aware of all options that are legally available to them in the country in which we practise if requested, following counselling by ourselves and our midwifery colleagues.

A senior colleague who influenced me greatly believed strongly that the whole area of testing and screening the fetus before birth should most definitely be an issue for discussion and decision-making between the obstetrician, midwife and parents alone. Sadly, today it sometimes seems that everyone else outside that triumvirate also has a view on how other people should live their lives. Live and let live is a maxim that could usefully be adopted by many people that I have come in contact with over the years.

Of course the issues around screening and pregnancy are incredibly emotive and we are all are entitled to hold and to develop a point of view. And it is important that those views are regularly reviewed and, where necessary, updated in the light of new evidence presented within a legal and appropriate moral and ethical framework. It is right, indeed you could say it is an obligation, for us all to try and convince our fellow citizens of the logic behind our own stance at any particular time in an orderly fashion. What we cannot do, though, what no one can or should do, is make judgements about a legally sound decision made by any fellow citizen unless we have walked a mile in their shoes. No one can fully understand and appreciate a personal situation unless they have experienced it themselves.

Every parent hopes to have to make as few difficult decisions as possible during pregnancy, and as clinicians, the fewer we have to have to address with parents the better. At the start of my career in the early 1970s, antenatal care was mainly about ensuring that the mother was as healthy as possible, and remained so throughout her pregnancy, and about preparing her for labour. The baby was simply considered to be an extension of the mother. No one knew the sex or approximate weight of the baby, its state of health or even, sometimes, what way round it was lying, until it was delivered.

There will be those reading this who yearn for a return to those days. 'What you don't know can't hurt you' is an expression that was often used – incorrectly I believe – to reassure parents. Having witnessed the advances in obstetrics over the past forty years and the accompanying improvements in prenatal screening and diagnosis, I fundamentally believe that the more we can find out – preferably non-invasively – before birth about the consequences of that birth for all involved, the better. Of course, what one does with the information gathered is something else entirely, but I have rarely, if ever, encountered a situation in which parents have regretted being informed in advance about an abnormal condition affecting their baby.

For example, in the pre-ultrasound days, a mother came in one night at term. She was in labour and as the midwife went to examine her, the membranes around the baby ruptured and the baby's umbilical cord, rather than the baby's head, suddenly appeared at the opening to the birth canal. The cord was pulsating well and all of us felt that it was extremely fortuitous that this event had occurred on a quiet Saturday night in the labour ward, which was fully staffed with a team who could perform a Caesarean section in a flash. We prepared the mother for this procedure, and five minutes after she became unconscious, we delivered her baby with an even stronger pulse. However, what we didn't know at the outset of the operation, and the mother didn't know as she went off to sleep full of expectation, was that the baby had anencephaly, a condition that meant that its brain had not developed beyond its anatomical base. Otherwise, the baby was perfect but it was incapable of any prolonged life after birth.

As the mother came round from her surgery and the anaesthetic, not only did she discover the terrible news about her baby, but she had also undergone an operation that would impact on her future reproductive life. So I am very much in favour of knowing what can be known. The basis of all medicine requires ideally, first and foremost, a clear diagnosis, for it is only with such a clinical opinion that plans can be considered and then implemented.

The introduction of ultrasound scanning means that this type of incident is highly unlikely to occur nowadays. Most major anatomical abnormalities can now be identified before birth when a good ultrasound machine is used by a trained sonographer on a mum with a baby lying in the normal position at the correct time of pregnancy. As well as looking at major organs and outlines, we also now increasingly refer to the observation of 'markers' or 'variants' when examining ultrasound images. Markers are ultrasound findings that identify one particular baby as being a little different from the majority. In themselves, markers do not indicate abnormalities per se. There are dozens of markers to observe, and it has been calculated that while as many as 50 per cent of all pregnancies have one marker, the vast majority (95 per cent) of babies are born without problems. We also know, however, that babies with major structural genetic abnormalities often also display ultrasonically detectable markers before the anomaly itself ever becomes obvious. Markers can therefore be pointers towards a greater underlying issue, indicating an increased risk of a mother having a baby with a certain abnormality. And it is this word 'risk' that brings on the myriad fears and anxieties that obstetricians want their patients to avoid.

Women throughout the developed world, and indeed the under-resourced world, are very aware that as they become older they are more likely, for example, to give birth to a baby with a chromosomal abnormality such as Down's Syndrome. My colleagues and I have often been fascinated by the way in which 'risk' is made an issue for mothers in many cultures when they get to the age of thirty-five. Certainly, over the last forty years, society has succeeded in making women of a certain age aware that they are at 'increased risk'. It wasn't until the late 1960s and early 1970s that it became possible to diagnose chromosomal abnormalities antenatally. This diagnosis was made possible using a procedure called an amniocentesis, whereby a doctor inserts a needle into the uterus and withdraws fluid from around the baby. That fluid contains live cells that have been shed from the fetal skin, and so can be cultured in the laboratory for three weeks, and then observed microscopically for their structure. Thus three weeks after the procedure, the parents can be informed of the exact chromosomal status of their baby.

In the late 1960s the British government did a cost analysis on the economic advantages of offering this amniocentesis to mothers in the UK. They came up with the statistic that, if the calculated risk of a mother having a baby with Down's Syndrome was one in two hundred, then there was a cost benefit to offering that mother an amniocentesis. That risk of one in two hundred occurs at the maternal age of thirty-seven. Hence, since 1969 or so, mothers aged thirty-seven and up have been made to feel that they are at a significantly higher risk. And of course they are. But they didn't *suddenly* become at risk. It's just that in 1969, it was considered economically viable to offer such women a test in the UK. In other words, if the risk of a certain pregnancy being so affected was one in one thousand (as it is at the age of thirty) then it would not have been economically viable to offer the test as the health economists of the time would compare the cost of offering this test to all women of that age to the cost to the state of caring for a child with Down's Syndrome and find that the former was higher. If they offered the test to women aged forty (risk one in one hundred) it would be of economic benefit. This is where the whole risk story really started, and I have always been fascinated that no matter where I have gone in the world, be it Belfast, Birmingham, Botswana or Bangkok, the definition of 'high risk' is the one calculated by the UK government in the late 1960s!

Of course two major issues have changed radically since those days. For a start, people with Down's Syndrome are now fully integrated into many societies and are not institutionalised as they often used to be. Second, diagnostic testing for Down's Syndrome is quite different from the testing that was carried out in the 1960s. While performing culture of fetal cells obtained by amniocentesis or indeed placental biopsy (chorionic villus sampling), we now have access to what is known as a FISH test which tells us within forty-eight to seventy-two hours whether the fetus in question has one of the three major chromosomal anomalies. Indeed, at the time of writing, it is now possible to completely non-invasively test a sample of blood from the mother at just ten weeks gestation and within a matter of days be informed with almost 100 per cent accuracy that the baby doesn't have one of the three major chromosomal abnormalities. The fact that chromosomal status can be detected without direct risk to the fetus is an enormous breakthrough for those of us who work in the field. This is very new technology, and will come at a price, at least in the short term. It will also, I imagine, open up an extensive and very necessary practical, moral, fiscal and ethical conversation at many levels in the years to come.

Meanwhile, from my own experience, I know that I could tell one woman of, say, forty-seven that there was a one in ten chance that her baby could have abnormal chromosomes, and she could say to me, 'Are you telling me doctor that if I had ten babies, only one of them would have this problem? Well that's good enough for me.' And yet the response of a twenty-five-year-old, whose risk of having a baby with Down's Syndrome is one in two thousand, could be, 'You mean it could happen to me?'

In thinking about the issue of risk, I always remember the writings of journalist John Diamond who, before his far too early death from cancer in 2001, wrote about his experience of the disease. In his book *C: Because Cowards Get Cancer Too* he told the story of how his wife, Nigella Lawson, went for an ultrasound scan when she was pregnant with their daughter Cosima. The scan picked up small cysts on the baby's brain, these markers being indicators of a possible chromosomal abnormality. In a state of shock the couple went to the fetal medicine department where a doctor talked to them about 'a fetal blood test with a 1 in 100 chance of inducing miscarriage balanced against the 1 in 250 chance that the cysts indicated something nasty'. John goes on to make the point that as soon as a patient hears the word risk, that risk effectively becomes 50/50. The listening patient is almost oblivious to any other calculations presented to them. For a parent considering what the particular risks are of their baby having a certain condition, it comes down to one thing: the baby has it, or it doesn't. This is what goes on in the mind of most parents when given any risk odds that are accompanied by the words 'increased' or 'high'.

My own approach when it comes to prenatal screening and counselling has always been to ask the mother whether, if she was making a bet, she would want to know the odds or the facts. If she wanted facts, then she was better to have a diagnostic test, such as an amniocentesis or similar test that, while potentially invasive, provided a diagnosis. More often than not, I found that women wanted facts and that it was far more important for them to know the answer to questions such as 'How good is that operator at putting a needle in my uterus?' or 'What are the obstetrician's success rates and miscarriage rates?' Those are the key questions that parents need answered.

Interestingly, in many countries in Europe, such as France for example, women of all ages often present themselves for an amniocentesis in the first instance. One might be tempted to imagine that these women are only interested in identifying abnormalities so that they may proceed to termination, but they are not. They simply want the facts, a diagnosis, and to be able to plan from there. I remember reading that in one of the Nordic countries, of women who are provided with a diagnosis confirming that their baby has Down's Syndrome, for example, 50 per cent proceed to termination of pregnancy, on the basis that they are not equipped with the mental resilience to continue with the pregnancy. The other 50 per cent take the diagnosis on board and prepare for the birth of a baby with Down's Syndrome. This is a refreshing approach.

As an obstetrician, you have to adapt to each patient who comes through the door of your consultation room, but you can't help being affected by what people say to you over the years. At the start of my career as a consultant I was asked to speak to a local group of parents and their children who all had one thing in common. They all had a child or a sibling with spina bifida, a condition in which the covering of the spinal cord is incomplete and which can result in varying degrees of motor loss and function, and, at times, mental impairment. I explained to the group the methods available for screening across the UK at that time. I seemed to get an unusually and unexpectedly warm reception, and this comfortable ambience continued over tea and biscuits afterwards. I spoke to one man who was there with his eighteen-year-old daughter who was in a wheelchair. He thanked me very much for my talk and commented that his view was that it was about time that Northern Ireland came into line with the rest of the UK and offered screening for spina bifida. I shared his view, but said that I was perhaps mildly confused as it appeared to me that he had a fine daughter who he seemed to love dearly. Why would he desire not to repeat the experience I briefly wondered? He seemed to be of a very happy disposition, and I was a little surprised by his enthusiasm for screening. He looked me in the eyes and said, 'Aye right, doctor, but no one needs two.' He and his wife had decided, following the birth of two healthy children, and then the birth of a beloved daughter with spina bifida, that they didn't want to take the risk of having more children that would be at an increased risk of requiring medical and community intervention. For him the very idea of prenatal screening and diagnosis was a godsend. Others obviously have a different view, which is my point.

Robert and Eileen were a couple facing a dilemma when I

met them some years ago. When Eileen had her scan at eighteen weeks, several markers were identified. The couple wanted to know what this signified and, after consultation, we carried out an amniocentesis. The result came back as Trisomy 18, or Edwards Syndrome. This finding was a devastating blow to Robert and Eileen as it meant that it was extremely likely that the baby would die very shortly after birth. After a lot more counselling, and discussion with family and friends about their situation, Eileen and Robert felt that she was strong enough to 'let nature take its course' and continue with the pregnancy. I agreed with her decision. In my job, you can quite quickly determine who has the family support and personal tools to cope in a situation like this, and those who – while they might be extremely able in another situation – would struggle greatly to cope.

At or around term, Eileen went into spontaneous labour and delivered naturally a baby boy who had Edwards Syndrome. I went in to see her the next morning: the baby was still alive and she was nursing him. Sadly, he died less than a week later. I saw Robert and Eileen for a review six weeks after the birth. I will always remember what Eileen said at that meeting: 'Those five days were amongst the best ones of our lives.' I thought it was tremendous that she had possessed the mental resilience to carry on with the pregnancy and to prepare herself for the likely outcome, and it was especially wonderful that she had so many positive memories. When my first daughter was born, following many years of infertility, I remember looking at her in the cot when she was ten days old and thinking to myself that even if she died that night, no one could ever take those ten days away from me. Back in the 1970s early infant death was much more common and all of us young parents felt that quite keenly – everybody knew someone who had tragically suffered a cot death. We knew that awful things could happen. Tragic as they were for others, such deaths also prepared us in some ways for tragic outcomes to pregnancy. Nowadays, cot deaths are extremely rare, and so when a sudden explained or unexplained death does occur, it is especially lonely for the parents. They feel particularly isolated.

Did you know that a butterfly only lives a total of fourteen days? Amazing really when you think of all the skill and aerodynamic design that goes into one of nature's most beautiful creatures. And a pearl only exists because an oyster has been abnormally insulted by the introduction of a grain of sand into its shell. Without that grain of sand to irritate the oyster, the pearl would not exist. We are here in this world for only a fleeting moment and our impact on others cannot be measured in years, months and days.

A lofty suggestion

Some years ago I found myself in Hargeisa in Somaliland with a team of healthcare workers from the UK and Ireland. We were working with a local Somaliland faculty – led by the indomitable and inspiring midwife, politician and hospital CEO Edna Ismail – to provide Emergency Obstetric Life-saving Skills courses to help address the tragic loss of mothers and babies in pregnancy and childbirth in that amazing country. These courses address the ten most common causes of maternal and newborn death. No hi-tech apparatus is required to deliver them, just men and women of goodwill, knowledge and good spirit willing to get on a plane and to go and meet up for a few days with their healthcare counterparts in the under-resourced world. It's been proven that these courses save lives.

In Somaliland we had wonderful multimedia commun-ications, and could use email and mobile phones. We showed PowerPoint presentations, and had hands-on digital interactive teaching aids and online care assessments to help us communicate, but we were in a country without proper roads. We travelled on tracks that were a system of potholes connected by deep ruts.

We had one afternoon off during our trip, and were taken by our hosts to a recently discovered cave with animal images on the wall that were painted some twenty thousand years ago. It was clear to me that humankind's ability and desire to communicate is only curtailed by the limits of imagination, resources and effort. Even all those years ago, people realised the importance of communicating with those around them, and with future generations.

The majority of women in the world deliver their babies without any trained personnel at their side. When a woman is in labour, and things are not going to plan, the outcome for that pregnancy depends almost entirely on the mother's ability to make contact with personnel that can make a difference. First, of course, the mother needs to recognise that there is a problem or, if she lacks the knowledge to do this, then she needs to have a birth attendant who is appropriately equipped to know when something is amiss.

It sounds simple, but whether we are referring to rural Africa or a brand new maternity unit in any city, delay in diagnosis, delay in getting the patient to the correct area, and delay in getting the appropriate personnel to that bedside and instigating appropriate management strategies can have tragic and devastating consequences. Good communication systems are essential to the provision of good healthcare.

Back in the 1970s, the majority of the mothers attending our hospital in Belfast did not have phones in their houses, never mind their pockets, and certainly did not have access to a family car. If transport was required during the day, people relied on buses and taxis; at night the only options tended to be a friend's car, taxis or ambulances.

Well-educated mothers very often quickly know when something is wrong in their pregnancy and, when they need to get to hospital, they and their family tend to think and act fast. Mothers have an inherent ability to recognise when all is not well and this instinct, when combined with the advice given during antenatal classes, means that most women know when to get concerned. 'Always listen to what women have to say as they are rarely incorrect' is a good maxim for those working in our speciality, especially given the fact that when pregnancies run into difficulties, things tend to get serious very quickly.

In the 1970s and 1980s, Belfast suffered from an additional

problem when it came to mothers getting to hospital to give birth. The Troubles were at their height and it wasn't always safe or practical to venture out at night and the likelihood of getting anywhere fast was slim. The ambulance service did its best in the most difficult circumstances, but their vehicles were, and sadly still are, often a target for unruly mobs who seem to equate a uniform with authority, and therefore see them as fair game for a pelting as they drive down the road on an emergency.

When I started in obstetrics in the 1970s there had recently been a few medical tragedies and near misses in the Belfast area, primarily because of poor communication and because those in need had been unable to obtain appropriate transport to hospital. This had a knock-on effect for those providing healthcare. In Belfast maternity units, for example, there developed a very liberal approach to induction of labour at or around term (forty weeks), so that mothers would be able to leave their homes in an orderly fashion and be delivered during daylight hours.

This kind of approach wasn't ideal: some women were induced a bit too early as we weren't that smart at knowing exactly when term was and – as we weren't that slick at induction itself in those days – the whole procedure got a pretty bad name. Labours were often very prolonged and hard, with no epidurals, but the majority of mothers were much happier to be in the relative safety of the maternity unit at 3 a.m. in the morning, rather than searching for a working phone box out on the street.

The National Health Service was set up to give people of all backgrounds and social classes access to warm, clean, friendly wards with excellent nursing and all appropriate treatments available to them. In recent times, however, it has been struggling to provide a first-class service on a third-class ticket. Back in the early days, just after the NHS had been set up, my predecessors in obstetrics and midwifery were dealing with a population of fairly young women who often had a number of young children at home, and a husband out working during the day. Although many women with health problems did spend large parts of their pregnancies in hospital, the aim was to have as few women as possible doing so – women were needed at home to care for their children.

Antenatal care had to be tailored to suit the social circumstances of the time and this often meant that patients with even potentially high-risk clinical situations that were temporarily dormant, could be allowed to return home on condition that they might have to come back in quickly, and that they would be able to do so. This way of working was demonstrated to me for the first time during a ward round with the consultant Gavin Boyd at the Royal Maternity Hospital. I was one of ten medical students standing around the bed of Rose Lavery who lived in one of the many housing estates situated close to the hospital. Her husband, who had been unemployed for a number of years, had just recently got a job. She had three children already (aged seven, five and three), was at thirty-three weeks gestation, and had been admitted with slight vaginal bleeding. Fairly state-of-the-art early ultrasound had suggested that the placenta might be in front of the baby's head, but there was no definitive diagnosis. Clinically Mr Boyd was sceptical of the results of the scan, as shortly after admission the bleeding had settled and Mrs Lavery was now 'stable'. This was fair enough, certainly in 1972. Ultrasound was in its infancy and Mr Boyd, an experienced consultant, was very sceptical of these 'newfangled toys' that were trying to replace common sense and centuries of clinical nous.

Mr Lavery, and indeed Mrs Lavery, were putting Mr Boyd under huge pressure to allow the latter to go home. On reflection, I find it fascinating that – although there were no locks on the doors of the wards – patients never, certainly in 1972, just walked out of the hospital without the consent of the medical or midwifery staff. In those days, if a patient wanted to leave the hospital against medical advice, they had to sign an AMA (Against Medical Advice) form saying that they accepted responsibility for the consequences of discharging themselves. I think these forms are now obsolete, but I was always amazed that patients who had decided to discharge themselves agreed to sign the form, no matter how determined, angry or forceful they were.

Mrs Lavery was certainly not the type of person to think of discharging herself, but she was keen to get back to her house and her children. In the Belfast urban environment women often didn't move far from the family home when they got married, so there were always parents and in-laws to help out with family matters.

The big question to be answered around the bed that day regarding Mrs Lavery was whether it would be safe for Mr Boyd to allow her to go home for the time being. It was our very first obstetric ward round and Mr Boyd was keen that we should learn how to take a relevant history from a patient. One of my student colleagues, George Rodgers was asked by Mr Boyd to take it in this particular case. George turned to Mrs Lavery and started thus, 'Mrs Lavery, could you tell me when your last menstrual period was?' Mrs Lavery was about to answer, when Mr Boyd interrupted, 'No, no, no, don't be asking her that at this stage, ask her where she lives.' George then asked her where she lived and was given the answer. She apparently lived on the edge of a housing estate about four miles away on up the Falls Road. Mr Boyd then said, 'Okay, what's the next question you are going to ask her?' George again proffered the question, 'When was your last menstrual period?' Again Mr Boyd interrupted, 'No, no, no, ask her if she has a phone.' George then asked her if she had a phone, to which Mrs Lavery replied, 'A phone? Don't be daft, we only just got a television.'

Mr Boyd then looked at George and said, 'What are you going to ask her now?' George turned again to Mrs Lavery and said, 'When was your last menstrual period?' Now, it is only fair to interrupt at this stage to offer some support for George. We had been instructed at the start of our course that when taking a history from a maternity patient, the first question we should ask was 'When was your last menstrual period?' as almost all decisions in pregnancy were directly related to the gestation of the pregnancy in question. George was correct to ask the question but it was a touch inappropriate in these circumstances to keep persevering when it was pretty obvious that Mr Boyd clearly had more practical details at the forefront of his mind. Again, George was interrupted by Mr Boyd who said, 'No, no, no, why don't you ask her if there is a telephone box at the bottom of the street?' George turned to Mrs Lavery and asked, 'Is there a telephone box at the bottom of the street?' Mrs Lavery informed him that there was, but that the receiver had been ripped off and there wasn't a pane of glass left in it. Again, Mr Boyd looked at George, more in hope than expectation and beckoned him to ask the next question. George asked, 'When was your last menstrual period?' Again Mr Boyd interrupted him and said, 'No, no, no, ask her does she have access to transport?' George asked Mrs Lavery if she had access to transport and she said, 'Not at all, my husband's brother has a van from work, but he lives in Antrim, twenty-five miles away.' Mr Boyd said, 'Right, Mr Rodgers, we have to find out how Mrs Lavery is going to communicate with us if we let her go home. What question are you going to ask her that would resolve this issue once and for all, and please don't ask her when her last menstrual period occurred.'

None of us knew what George was going to come out with but he certainly changed the mood around that four-bedded bay when he said, 'Mrs Lavery, tell me, does your husband keep pigeons?'

Hold your tongue till you're sure

In recent decades medical practitioners have begun to communicate with and counsel patients and relatives much more than they used to. In the past, doctors could often get away with saying very little. Better indeed, some would say, to keep your mouth closed and be thought of as a fool, rather than opening your mouth and proving it.

I once worked with a consultant who, having obtained a history and performed a careful examination and thorough investigation, would carefully make a differential diagnosis in his mind and then form an action plan. He would communicate none of this to the patient in question. Rather, he would quite simply look at her and say, 'I am bringing you in on Tuesday, and you let me do the worrying.' Many of his patients were very, very happy with this approach, such was their total faith in his ability. From my own observations, his method, despite its lack of dialogue, had much to recommend it, as was evidenced by his happy patients.

Many consultants in the past also felt it was inappropriate to become too close to patients either emotionally or even physically during examination, believing that to do so was a recipe for disaster. One consultant took this a bit too seriously, and before the start of his surgical outpatient clinic on a Monday morning, he got the nursing sister in charge to securely tie the plastic chair earmarked for the patient to the radiator at the back of the room with the use of binding twine. The consultant then sat behind his desk at the other end of the room.

This no-touch technique could also be used when it came to the physical examination. A mid-twentieth-century respiratory consultant of note had a special stethoscope with a six-foot length of tubing that he used when doing his rounds in public wards at the time when tuberculosis was rife. He would instruct the nurse to hold the bell end of the stethoscope on the patient's chest while he stood in relative safety at some distance behind the curtain surrounding the bed. He further endeavoured to ensure his own safety by instructing the patient to 'cough towards the nurse, my good man'.

My own generation, however, is a little different. We tend to share many of our clinical deliberations with those in our care, and thus often take the patient with us on the clinical journey to arriving at a diagnosis.

One evening in 1981, one of my junior registrar colleagues, Charlie, was called to casualty to see an apparently acute clinical case. The casualty officer was examining an eighteen-year-old girl called Patricia with a mass, or large bump, rising from her pelvis. When the casualty officer saw her in the casualty cubicle, she was obviously in desperate pain and distress. He reckoned it was pretty obviously a maternity complication and was therefore outside his realm of specialisation, and so he had urgently called one of our team to assist. Charlie went to see the patient and found her to be otherwise stable, apart from the pretty obvious pregnancy. Patricia's mother, who had come to the hospital with her daughter, was asked to leave the cubicle and Charlie got on with his assessment of the situation, which included palpating the 'bump' in question. He swiftly presented Patricia with his working diagnosis: that she was six months pregnant and was having a complication, 'maybe even with twins'. The day before, Charlie had seen his first case of 'Twin to Twin Transfusion Syndrome' and he reckoned that this was another case. This syndrome occurs when two fetuses share one placenta: one twin becomes a donor and the other twin a recipient. The recipient can get an acute increase in fluid volume around it, which can cause great pain to the mother because of increased abdominal swelling.

Patricia was indignant and forcefully denied all likelihood of pregnancy, or even the possibility that she had ever had sex. But Charlie pushed his point: 'Well listen, these situations don't occur just by kissing, we are going to have to tell your mother what the problem is. It is better to confide in me and I can help to break the ice for you.' Charlie was a very caring and thoughtful person, but he felt that the sooner Patricia owned up, the sooner action could be taken to address the clinical problem. Patricia said, 'But doctor, Seamie promised me that I wouldn't get pregnant and we only did it once.' Charlie assured Patricia that she wasn't unique among the teenage population in Belfast at that time and further promised her that he would speak to her mother and do his best to smooth things over once he had delivered the news. Charlie slipped outside and found Patricia's mother. 'Mrs Hill,' he said, 'as far as I can see the problem is that your daughter has a pretty rare complication of pregnancy, but Patricia herself will be fine.' Mrs Hill was flabbergasted. 'That's impossible – she can't be pregnant. She promised me she wasn't having sex.'

Charlie and the mother both went back in to see Patricia, and the mother displayed huge sympathy and compassion for her daughter who was in such agony, but was also obviously angry about her daughter's pregnancy.

Charlie slipped out of the cubicle in order to make arrangements with the ambulance team to transfer the patient to the maternity department. While on the phone, he was not surprised to overhear Mrs Hill saying, 'You might think I am angry, but just you wait and see what happens when your daddy finds out.' This threat of the potential reaction from the other parent is one used in many situations in childhood. I've used it myself with my kids. However, when it comes to maternity matters I have often observed that a father's reaction to the apparent bad news is often totally the opposite to what the girls have been prepared for or worried about. There were many times that a single girl in my care would, after being given the diagnosis of an unexpected and unplanned pregnancy, respond by saying, 'My dad will go berserk. He'll throw me out of the house.' Rarely, if ever, did I actually see this happen. Indeed, handled carefully, the father will often relish the opportunity of being his daughter's protector. In my experience a father is more likely to respond to dynamite news with comments such as, 'It's not what you or I wanted at this time, but don't you worry. We will get through this together. Now let me give you a hug.' In reality, *this* would be the most common response I have witnessed over the past four decades and even if it's not the first reaction, it is usually the ultimate one.

Meanwhile, an ambulance arrived and all involved – Patricia, her mum and Charlie – went to the maternity unit, a hundred metres away. Charlie located the portable ultrasound machine, and while waiting for it to warm up, he applied some gel to Patricia's abdomen. By this time both Patricia and her mother were becoming excited about seeing the baby, or if Charlie's hunch was correct, babies. The time arrived: Charlie put the ultrasound scanner on Patricia's tummy and scanned every corner of her abdomen. He didn't speak for about thirty seconds, not because he was being careful about communication – it was a bit late for that – but because he saw pretty quickly that there was absolutely, positively and, devastatingly for Charlie, nothing inside Patricia's abdomen except for a very over-full bladder! Patricia had in fact developed an acute retention of urine and was not pregnant at all.

Charlie spent the next thirty seconds trying to get his story straight before he shared it with Patricia and her mum. The solution to the clinical problem was easy – simply catheterise the patient – but at what price to his credentials. Patricia had revealed intimacies that did not need to be revealed. Her mother had lost her temper with her and that need not have occurred. Charlie had lost face big time – but he had learnt a very important lesson the hard way. And as for as poor Seamie, he had probably done very little wrong at all, but had ended up being maligned anyway.

The diagnosis of successful pregnancy and the diagnosis of non-successful pregnancy are colossal for all concerned. For doctors and midwives it is imperative that when you give somebody good news, you are 100 per cent correct. If you are going to give them bad news, make sure you are 200 per cent correct. Perhaps the previous generation of doctors who kept much of their mental gymnastics and deliberations to themselves had a point. Once it's blurted out, or written down, it's a matter of material fact. And that can make for, at best, a sticky and, at worst, a devastating situation for all concerned.

Ah yes!

The association between anaesthetics and childbirth goes back to Victorian times. We are told in the Bible, the Koran and the Tanakh that the pain associated with childbirth is natural, and indeed, many religions have traditionally taken a very dim view of those who help to alleviate the suffering of mothers in labour. In the tenth century, for example, the Catholic church endorsed *Malleus Maleficarum* (or 'Hammer of the Witches'), a treatise on the prosecution of witches that led to many thousands of women, a significant number of them midwives, being branded witches and burned at the stake. Midwives were included as they were seen as being anti-church law in using their clinical skills to help mothers deal with pain during labour.

As a frequent visitor to Kruger National Park in South Africa, I have observed first-hand that wild animals experience virtually no pain when giving birth. They also appear to have evolved themselves quite nicely within their own particular species to a point where even a huge bear gives birth to a baby weighing on average only one kilogram! Domestication of a species seems to hold the key to producing problems in childbirth. Cows, sheep and horses often require the local veterinary surgeon, whereas lions, tigers and elephants seem to take giving birth in their stride.

When in 1847 James Young Simpson from Edinburgh introduced chloroform to help alleviate the pain of labour, he was lauded in many quarters – including by Queen Victoria who received it during two of her labours – but castigated in many more. Simpson started something that would change the world of obstetrics and midwifery forever, and that would make the leaders of the various religions reassess their rather narrow view of what their womenfolk should endure. Something of a revolution, if you will.

In my own working lifetime, the widespread introduction of epidurals has, to me at least, not only provided a wonderful tool that has enabled obstetricians and midwives to do a better job, but it has brought dignity to many women during labour. Before the widespread use of epidurals and spinal anaesthesia, mothers either had to get through labour supported by a combination of midwifery support, nitrous oxide inhalation (laughing gas), narcotics such as morphine or pethidine (Demerol in the US) and/or general anaesthetic. To use just the first two is what many women aspire to but sometimes this just isn't possible. Drugs have their place, but their effects and side effects are widespread, and include maternal drowsiness and incoherence. In addition, many of these drugs do cross the placenta, and the fetus can be a bit too sleepy immediately after birth when too many of them are administered.

General anaesthesia use, while relatively safe nowadays, used to be associated with increased risk in pregnancy. Dr Liam Donaldson, a recent Chief Medical Officer for England and Wales, has said that when he was born, in the early 1950s, 1 in 1,000 previously healthy British people died as a result of being given a general anaesthetic, whereas now, the number who die in this manner annually is tiny.

Before epidurals, a Caesarean section or difficult assisted delivery could only be performed with the assistance of an anaesthetist providing a general anaesthetic. Administering an anaesthetic is much like piloting an aeroplane in that the take-off and landing are crucial – the process of putting the patient under the anaesthetic and bringing them out again are key. Both the anaesthetist and the pilot can have performed in as varied a set of situations as possible, read as many books as exist, and have as many 'flying' hours under their belt as humanly feasible, but the unexpected can still catch them out.

Maureen Williams was twenty-three years old when I met her in the labour ward in which I was the senior registrar on duty. She had been admitted in spontaneous labour and was about five days past her expected date of confinement. Her husband was a jolly guy called Roy. Roy was a plumber by trade and since I had occasion to be in and out of Maureen's room quite a lot during her day in labour, he and I found much humour in comparing our jobs. He saw a lot in common in our working lives, and the way he put it that day, I couldn't disagree. We all built up a good relationship as the day progressed, but Maureen's labour was slow and it became fairly evident in the wee small hours that progress was about to grind to a halt. I won't tell you exactly what Roy said, but he suggested that there was a blockage in a main pipe, and I agreed. I decided that I should telephone the consultant on-call to discuss the case.

In those days it was always important, before the clinical events of the evening in the labour ward unfolded, to check to see which consultant was on call. When a problem occurred, the consultant on the other end of the phone would listen attentively to the synopsis of the clinical situation as we saw it, but after a while we got to know how to get whichever consultant it was to agree with our desired course of action. At least, that is, when they stayed awake. The story is told that one night one of my colleagues was giving a rather prolonged account to the consultant and paused at one point to get a reply. On hearing nothing, he turned round to the nursing sister on labour ward and said, 'I think the old bugger has fallen asleep,' to be followed immediately by the sound of his consultant gruffly saying, 'Wrong – the old bugger is not asleep, he is thinking.'

This particular night I really felt that Maureen had suffered enough. She seemed a strong and healthy woman who did not have had any particular physical problems of her own that would deter the normal transfer of a baby into this world. We often talked about the three Ps that enable trouble-free childbirth. Is the Passageway big enough? Is the Passenger's head too big or in the incorrect position? Are the Powers of the womb's muscles strong enough? It was my own feeling that despite excellent power and probably a fairly adequate passage, Maureen's passenger (the baby) was just too big and was lying in a suboptimal position in the birth canal. It is much easier to come into this world either looking sideways or down – not looking up which was the position that Maureen's baby had assumed.

I knew, however, that the consultant I was phoning was particularly conservative. It is much easier to sit comfortably at home and say, 'Leave her another few hours and if there is no progress do a Caesarean' than to have to walk into the room yourself and explain a further delay to the parents. I was, therefore, careful with what I said, while at the same time telling the truth, the whole truth and nothing but the truth. I explained to him that Mrs Williams had been in labour the whole day, which she had, and that there was no recent progress, and that her cervix was only about two thirds dilated despite the use of an Oxytocin drip (an intravenous infusion of a naturally occurring hormone that mostly helps to progress labour by strengthening the womb's muscle contractions and may lead to quicker dilation of the cervix, much loved by many obstetricians and midwives, but loathed by a vociferous minority of the latter who see it as unnatural and a medical intervention).

The consultant then, not unexpectedly, said to me, 'And what do you think we should do Jim?' I carefully answered, 'Well, I don't think she would come to any harm if we gave her another few hours and then I could examine her again.' He thought for a second and then said, 'No, I don't think you will gain anything by doing that. You have driven this process as far as it will go. I would suggest you do a Caesarean section now.' Yes! I thought to myself, just the answer I wanted. This particular consultant always enjoyed showing his power by suggesting the opposite management strategy to the one we junior doctors put forward. He fell into the trap yet again!

Buoyed up with the news, I went to see Roy and Maureen and the relief all round was tremendous. The midwives too were delighted as they could see that Maureen could take no more. Watching a team in action, especially when that action is really required, is a joy to behold. I remember Roy commenting to me as we went into theatre that he had been well impressed by how everybody had very quickly and efficiently prepared his wife for surgery.

Roy waited in the fathers' room and we all trooped into theatre. I noted that the time was 4 a.m. Everybody that needed to be there was assembled. The senior registrar in anaesthetics was a good friend, and we had frequently been on night duty together and trusted each other. The sister in labour ward was a gem, the sort you never disagreed with, rather than the sort that you didn't dare to disagree with. The paediatrician had been called, just in case there were any problems with the baby after the birth. Everybody in the theatre was prepped and ready to go.

Just before the anaesthetic was given, the midwifery sister came forward and listened to the baby's heartbeat one more time in order to reassure us all that we could take our time and go steadily. I always thought this was a very onerous task. What if she got it wrong and we really ought to be rushing? Interestingly, I never saw this happen. Good midwives are the salt of the earth.

The induction of anaesthesia went well and Maureen was soon unconscious. We proceeded to do the Caesarean section and there were absolutely no problems doing surgery. A very well grown baby girl was delivered in good time. In those days, when the baby came out, it was mandatory to use a little vacuum pump to suck out the back of the baby's throat to clear it of secretions. Junior doctors and midwives got into serious trouble if they didn't do this. Nowadays they'd be in serious trouble if they did. Current thinking is that these natural secretions are best left where they are as they can be rich in constituents that help breathing. Also overly vigorous sucking of the back of the baby's throat can cause its heart rate to slow by excessive stimulation of the vagus nerve that runs in the tissues at this anatomical point. Another example of a 180-degree turn in medicine.

However, despite careful sucking and drying of the baby, she seemed almost lifeless – even though she had a good heart rate, she wasn't even taking a gasp. I quickly handed the baby over to the paediatricians and they laid her down in a Johnson cot equipped with a warm overhead light to try to keep her temperature at 37 degrees centigrade. The paediatricians immediately started bagging the baby with oxygen – putting a rubber mask over the baby's nose and mouth and encouraging the passage of pure oxygen into the baby's lungs – and reported very quickly that her heart rate and colour were good, but that she was making no effort to breathe.

This came as a huge shock to us as we had been carrying out the Caesarean section because of an apparent 'cephalopelvic disproportion' problem, rather than any fetal distress. Also, we had been reassured at the start of the procedure that the heartbeat was good, and I knew that the baby's umbilical cord was pumping regularly when I had delivered her. When things go wrong, one can't help going through the various possible explanations, and wondering if something has been missed. We all discussed the clinical possibilities but we could think of nothing that accounted for the baby's condition.

At least the baby was a good colour, and that was very important, but we were all terribly worried. Had the baby been lacking oxygen for some time? Was she lacking oxygen now? Maybe the baby had been subjected to an antenatal insult earlier in the pregnancy that was just manifesting itself now? All I could do was finish the Caesarean section. The anaesthetist had temporarily gone over to help the paediatrician. The paediatrician had called in his consultant colleague, but meanwhile the anaesthetist very slickly intubated the baby's trachea to enable mechanical ventilation. He passed a small tube into the baby's larynx so that direct ventilation of the baby's lungs could be achieved.

The paediatrician was now bagging the baby to keep her respiration going. The mood in the theatre had changed dramatically from the usual one of professional good nature to one of colossal concern. Having put in the last stitch and done a final instrument check, I looked over to the baby and saw that the situation was unchanged. I knew that I'd soon have to go out and tell Roy what was happening and also Maureen when she came round from her anaesthetic. While I was considering this, the anaesthetist said to me, 'Jim, I don't know what's going on here but I can't get Maureen to breathe by herself. I am going to have to leave the tube down.' If it was possible, everybody in theatre went even quieter.

Maureen's tracheal ventilation tube was reconnected to the ventilator. Again everything seemed to be normal – all her vital observations were exactly within normal limits, she didn't have a temperature, her pupils reacted to light, her blood pressure was normal, her pulse was normal, and the oxygen content of the peripheral circulation was normal. What the hell was going on?

We worked away with both the mother and the baby for some time and everybody went through the various factors that could be causing one or other, or indeed both situations. We knew that occasionally the stress of an anaesthetic could cause damage to a mother's brain and that thought crossed our minds. Again, I was thinking about what we would tell Roy if that turned out to be the situation?

Meanwhile, the anaesthetist had decided that the situation couldn't continue as it was, and he rang the consultant from the Intensive Care Unit in the nearby Royal Victoria Hospital. He came back in from the phone and said, 'They have agreed to take her over, and the ambulance will be here soon.' It was time to face Roy. I got a latest update from the paediatrician and the anaesthetist – there was no change. Both of them were definitely confused, albeit in a holding pattern since both the patients were clinically stable.

I went out to see Roy with a heavy weight of responsibility on my shoulders. 'Roy, things haven't gone exactly the way we had intended. Maureen is over the operation and it went well. The baby was delivered safely and both Maureen and your little daughter are pink but neither will breathe by themself. Maureen is going to be moved over to the Intensive Care Unit in the Royal and the baby is going to go back to the nursery here. They are both on breathing machines at the moment. To be honest with you, Roy, we just don't know what is going on. Why don't you come into theatre with me to see them?'

I wasn't sure myself whether the last idea was the right thing to have suggested or not, but I have found that sometimes seeing reality is better than imagining it, as quite often the mind can make things seem worse than they really are. Roy didn't crumble or overreact, but just stood firmly, stoically and listened intently.

We walked into the theatre, which was just across the corridor. The theatre was as bright as usual and as tidy as any theatre would look after surgery had been performed. Maureen was lying on the operating table and the corrugated bag of the respirator was going up and down about twenty times per minute. Just to the left of her was the Johnson cot with the baby lying on her back with the paediatrician blowing oxygen and air into her lungs around twenty times per minute. I felt an awful pain for Roy and what he must have been feeling as he faced this scene.

Roy looked at the whole scenario, looked at the anaesthetist, looked at his wife, looked at the paediatrician, looked at his newborn daughter and then looked at me and said, 'Ah yes, I'll tell you what it is, it's scoline apnoea, just like her sister!' My anaesthetic colleagues had already entertained the possibility of this exceedingly rare diagnosis, but I had thought it was inappropriate to share too many technicalities with Roy in the initial phase. But Roy came to the diagnosis immediately.

Scoline apnoea is a condition whereby the patient has a deficiency of the particular enzyme that breaks down the scoline that is given by the anaesthetist to temporarily stop spontaneous respiration so that the anaesthetist can take control when putting the patient asleep. The scoline should wear off rapidly, but with scoline apnoea this doesn't happen and the effects take some time to wear off. Exactly the same thing had happened to Maureen's sister a couple of years before, but for one reason or another, that information had not been passed on to us – the problem obviously ran in the family. The relief in the room was palpable. Case solved. Who said plumbing is easy?

A life saved

One view of doctors held by the general public is that we spend our time saving lives, and I suppose there is some truth to that perception. Those times when I have responded to an emergency and saved a life have been exhilarating and are imprinted on my mind forever.

One such occasion occurred very early on in my career. I was a houseman in the baby unit of the Jubilee Maternity Hospital and part of my remit was to be present at high-risk deliveries to administer resuscitative measures to newborn babies if necessary.

I have seen many changes in obstetrics in the last forty years, but one of the most startling is how rarely, nowadays, truly intensive resuscitative measures are required in the minutes after birth compared to how frequently this intervention was required in the 1970s. Back then, when an emergency delivery was being planned, whether by forceps or Caesarean section, we juniors would be summoned to appear at the labour ward at a moment's notice to join the midwives and the obstetricians who were already there. In the minutes prior to the imminent and urgent birth, I would prepare myself for all possible eventualities, such as the baby at birth being anything from apparently lifeless, with a slow or unrecordable heart rate and making no effort to breathe, to a vigorously crying baby who surprises everyone in the room by being unexpectedly healthy. Back then, the standard first steps taken to resuscitate someone were the ABC of Airway, Breathing and Circulation, and are as valid now as they were then. With nervous anticipation I would set out instruments and drugs ready for the arrival of the worst scenario: a 'flat baby', which was a baby that was often apparently lifeless with just a weak pulse to signal that resuscitation was possible, feasible and hopefully worthwhile.

I am told that in the 1960s and before, it was very rare to see a paediatrician at a delivery as resuscitative measures were traditionally left to the obstetrician and the midwife. Paediatricians tended to stay in the nursery and were presented with the clinical 'aftermath'. This led to paediatricians blaming any problems that arose on the obstetricians and midwives. I am told there was a fair amount of 'Well, the baby was all right when we gave it to you' from the obstetricians, and also an equal amount of 'Well, we got the baby in very poor condition and could only do our best'. The creation in the late 1960s of the job of perinatal paediatrician, a doctor who not only attended births but also specialised in care of the newborn, revolutionised care for babies. The main aim of any delivery up until that time was to make sure that the mother survived the labour, and was able to become pregnant again. The baby just had to take its chances. In order to try to improve the care given to babies at birth, a very famous international paediatrician, Dr Virginia Apgar, devised a system for assessing the state of the newborn as far back as 1952. That system is still in general use today worldwide. She asserted that new babies should be evaluated in five key areas – colour, tone, breathing effort, heart rate and reflex response – at intervals of a few minutes. The first readings are taken one minute after birth, and the baby is given a score of between zero and two in each category. These assessments are repeated again, five minutes after birth and then ten minutes after birth and the scores added together to give a total out of ten. It is universally recognised that babies, for example, who have Apgar scores of less than 6 at five minutes have a guarded prognosis, though there are myriad stories of geniuses that started life with much lower scores.

Prior to her death, Dr Apgar revealed that the main reason she invented the score was to 'try to get the paediatrician to not just come to the labour ward, but to stay for more than ten seconds'. Before the Apgar score was introduced, it was fairly commonplace for a paediatrician on call, on being urgently summoned to the delivery room, to stick his or her head around the door, and if s/he heard crying, immediately to close the door again and leave. As I have said, relationships between obstetricians and paediatricians in the mid-twentieth century certainly were frequently fraught, but are now perfect, at least in the environment in which I was privileged to work.

While resuscitation of a newborn was, and is, feasible in a well-prepared environment when I was a houseman, we sometimes had to make do in unusual circumstances. Working in the same unit as me in 1974 was a senior house officer in obstetrics, Tony Traub. He graduated a year ahead of me and lived next door, and we often spent the early part of our evenings, on the days neither of us were on call, chatting over the fence about the events of our working day. While I was a houseman in the baby unit and before I started obstetrics, he would tell me of his high-risk deliveries in the labour ward and I would tell him of my apparent heroics and resuscitation efforts with babies.

One day though, we unexpectedly got the opportunity to work together. A normal ambulance had been called to the home of a young girl of fourteen who had been off school for some days with abdominal cramps. The ambulance men discovered her on the floor and clutching her abdomen in extreme agony with what seemed to be pretty obvious colic. She was quickly transported to Belfast City Hospital, which was ten minutes away. As they turned into the hospital grounds, the ambulance man who was sitting with the young girl suddenly noticed the foot of a baby protruding from beneath her clothing. He quickly told his colleague not to turn left for casualty, but to turn right for the maternity unit.

When they got there, the men swiftly unloaded the trolley from the back of the ambulance and wheeled it into the ground floor of the Jubilee Maternity Hospital with the intention of going up in the lift to the labour ward. At exactly the same time Tony and I were just about to exit the lift to head home. When the lift doors opened we were greeted by the young girl in agony and two very concerned-looking ambulance men. A quick exchange of information occurred and a rapid examination revealed that a term-sized baby, presenting feet first, had been born right up to its chest. Very worryingly, the baby's chest was facing frontward. Left in this precarious position, the baby would not be delivered alive. A small portion of the umbilical cord was also visible, and it was beating, but only just.

Tony and I quickly introduced ourselves to the girl, whose name was Pauline, and took charge. Using one of the ambulance blankets to give him purchase on a rather slippery baby, Tony rapidly and expertly turned the baby around 180 degrees so that its back and not its chest was facing upwards. 'Hands off the breech' is the mantra taught to all obstetricians in normal circumstances but that really didn't apply here and Tony proceeded to do a beautifully executed breech extraction, bringing out the baby's left shoulder and then its right shoulder and then carrying out a Mauriceau-Smellie-Viet procedure with his left hand to deliver the baby's head.

When the baby came out, it was limp and lifeless and looked like it had a birth Apgar score of zero. Tony handed the baby to me and I set it on a blanket on the floor, still attached to its mother by the umbilical cord. The cord was barely pulsing. Using a finger wrapped in a blanket, I wiped the mucous and secretions from the baby's mouth. Then I immediately, and very gently, blew air into the baby's mouth using the mouth-to-mouth technique, while at the same time using two fingers to regularly press up and down in the middle of the chest with the intention of pumping blood around its little circulation system.

In the meantime, the ambulance staff had called the labour ward but, within a few minutes (though it felt like an hour), the baby was gasping by itself, its heart rate was up to 120 beats per minute and it was losing that pale, mottled look and was becoming pink and active. A quick glance at mum revealed her to be calm, having been very well attended by Tony and the paramedics. She was shocked, naturally, but at least the agony had disappeared. What had also disappeared was the cloak of silence in which she had shrouded her pregnancy. She had told no one that she was pregnant.

While we waited for an incubator to be brought down from the labour ward, Pauline's parents arrived. They had been following the ambulance in their car. You can imagine the look of shock on their faces when they saw that their daughter had given birth. But that shock was quickly followed by huge compassion and love as they embraced their daughter and new granddaughter. Love is indeed an incredible glue, and I am pretty sure that none of us ever forgot the scene in front of us that day.

It later transpired, as it does in many of these cases, that Pauline had realised that she was pregnant but had blocked the reality out of her mind, hoping it would go away. This was the 1970s and Pauline must have had a great fear of telling her parents that she was in the family way. Deep inside, these teenage mums must have felt very proud of themselves in achieving motherhood, but they often experienced a lot of negativity or, at best, mixed signals from those around them. Nowadays teenagers have more choices, but often still do choose to be mums before fully achieving maturity. Most people still don't think that being a mother at this stage is the best option, and on paper they might be correct, but I have been impressed by many of the teenage mums that I have treated and have found that they dealt with pregnancy, birth and the early days of parenthood responsibly and ably. Many teenage mums who remain single don't rush into a second pregnancy for at least a decade after the birth of their first child. They seldom declare regret about the first pregnancy, though they do confide that the 'growing up' period between adolescence and adulthood was, for them, accelerated exponentially.

I have no doubt that Pauline made a great mum, for she had

already learnt two important lessons: that things often don't work out as badly as you imagine, and that she was able to deal with all eventualities. Of course, while there are many planned and accidental teenage pregnancies nowadays, at least the teenager in question usually has fewer worries about the reaction at home. In contrast, Pauline was in fear of the consequences for her home life and adult life, the anticipated anger of her parents, the risk of being cast out from society and of being thrown out of the house throughout her pregnancy. In reality, all was fine, and the irony was that the very day that she gave birth, Pauline was due to be in school to receive a first prize in Home Economics and Childcare!

The last hours of that working day were full of powerful emotion for all involved: Pauline, her parents, the ambulance men and us. Birth has an incredibly uplifting effect most of the time, even if a pregnancy is not always planned, or even initially wanted. A newborn baby is almost invariably the catalyst for a cascade of love and positive emotion.

Selfish or sensible?

Many women, given the choice and having considered all the options, choose to have their baby delivered by Caesarean section, especially if they have already experienced that particular method of delivery.

When I started out as an obstetrician Caesarean sections were a method of delivery brought on by necessity rather than choice. A woman was often *in extremis* by the time an obstetrician made the decision to perform a Caesarean section, and there was a real sense of failure for the obstetrician at having to resort to that procedure. Add to that the genuine risks of general anaesthetic and open surgery in an already exhausted woman and you have a recipe for potential disaster.

In much of the world today women still have their Caesareans after fairly arduous and exhausting labours. Indeed while there are many who are unimpressed by the allegedly needlessly high rates for Caesareans in the resourced world, hundreds of thousands of mothers and babies die every year in the under-resourced world because they do not have access to that method of delivery. Approximately 30 per cent of women in the world have no antenatal care, 50 per cent of women give birth outside a birthing unit; and 50 per cent have no skilled birth attendant, nurse, midwife or doctor, with them at the time of delivery. It is no wonder that a mother dies in childbirth every minute of every day and that 95 per cent of maternal deaths occur outside birthing units. These are sobering facts, and sadly reflect the place of women in many societies. Their health and welfare are not priorities, and they are often considered to be easily replaceable. We have much rebalancing still to do in the international arena. Meanwhile, some people continue to use their energies to complain that too many women in the developed world have Caesareans, rather than using their influence to address the root causes of why women die in the under-resourced world.

Caesareans can often appear to be daunting albeit life-saving procedures, but nowadays, by and large, women in the resourced world do not have that same sense of foreboding when undergoing the operation as they might have had, say, in the 1970s. Anaesthetists are the main professional group we have to thank for this development as they have transformed both the risks and the experience. Historically, it was considered pretty dangerous to anaesthetise a pregnant woman. Until rather late in the twentieth century, mothers who needed Caesareans or potentially risky forceps deliveries required a general anaesthetic. Sounds simple, but in the case of a pregnant mum who needed an emergency intervention just after a large meal had been consumed, who also had a large womb and baby pressing on the diaphragm, the administration of an anaesthetic could be very difficult indeed. Now – and this has been the case for the past couple of decades – the vast majority of Caesareans are performed under regional spinal anaesthesia, allowing the mother to be totally compos mentis throughout the procedure, and the mother's partner to remain with her for the duration of the operation. Pain relief is given prophylactically and any nausea experienced post-operatively is quickly addressed. I once asked a mother under spinal anaesthesia if she was experiencing any discomfort, to which she replied, 'Not at all – it just feels like you are rummaging around in my shopping bag!' Most women who have a Caesarean in our part of the world do have a good experience. Indeed this may well be reflected in this country's medico-legal bill. About 50 per cent of all settlements in the NHS are for obstetric cases and 98 per cent of these are for women who did not have a Caesarean even though 25 per cent of women give birth by that method. Makes you stop and think.

Each year the government sets aside one thousand pounds for settlements for every pregnant mother unit, actuaries having calculated that down the line that will be the typical amount that will be required to pay the lawyers and the plaintiffs. Antenatal care, as presently provided, costs about sixty pounds per mother. Maybe some of this projected medico-legal bill could be used for a bit of forward planning that really improves the care of pregnant woman antenatally and in labour, by trying to prevent the cases that lead to large settlements. Most women do not have more than three babies so these pregnancies should be cared for by the best team available at every turn. That team should include, as a matter of course in all cases, senior midwives, obstetricians, anaesthetists and paediatricians working together, always with trainees, to make sure that every mum gets optimal care. I feel that there is too much emphasis put on the mother having a good experience rather than a safe one.

During my time in private practice I quickly realised that if you told a woman that everything is fine when you didn't know for sure, you were leaving yourself open to a huge loss of maternal confidence if anything went wrong. The raising of expectations for labour progress, for example, must be tempered with reality. We are constantly being encouraged to tell all our charges of the risks of interventions such as induction of labour, epidurals, forceps and Caesareans, yet there is no such imperative to inform them of the realistic outcomes of apparently normal labour at all!

My view is that there are too many experts out there involved in maternity care provision who haven't been in a labour ward since they were born, and who not only have views that are often diametrically opposed to those of the mother, but who are also in such public and professional positions that they can penalise the mother, mentally and physically, for having that alternate view. For example, the vast majority of Caesareans are performed for strong clinical indications, and only very few when the *only* indication is the mother's request. Yet this small group of mothers who request sections is often vilified in the media in a most unfair manner. A simple maternity mantra would be 'Don't criticise till you've walked a mile in her shoes.'

Although I don't know any obstetrician who would treat a woman differently depending on whether he or she saw her in an NHS setting or a private setting, this is certainly the perception amongst many of these vocal opinion setters, and therefore amongst mothers. Some mothers have been led to believe that they have to attend an obstetrician privately in order to have an elective Caesarean section, whether there is a weighty clinical indication or not.

At last, slowly and surely, opinion is settling down and the National Institute for Health and Clinical Excellence (NICE) has now accepted that, in England and Wales at least, a woman can opt for a Caesarean as long as all benefits and risks have been made clear to her, and after appropriate discussion and support from a healthcare professional. Until NICE came up with this sensible decision, women had to shop around to find a unit and team that would be sympathetic to her desires. Sometimes this meant travelling quite a distance. Some of us wonder for how long NICE's present logical and compassionate view will be sustained.

When Rosemary, pregnant with her second child, walked through the door of my consulting rooms and told me her story, my first thought was that she was subtly declaring a desire for a Caesarean section. In Rosemary's first pregnancy, she had absolutely no problems in becoming pregnant, remaining pregnant, being pregnant, starting labour, labouring, or delivering the baby's head. Indeed, everything had gone very well and to plan. When the baby's head was delivered, however, there was a problem getting the baby's shoulders out. This is known as shoulder dystocia, and can happen in any pregnancy, but it is more likely to happen with large babies. This is an emergency situation and can be very serious as it prevents the baby from breathing – the head is delivered but the chest is stuck inside. As this is an emergency, medical and midwifery staff must act quickly to get the baby out and this can occasionally cause harm.

Rosemary's baby was delivered within the appropriate length of time and in good condition, but its clavicle (or collar bone) had been broken during the delivery. It is difficult to prove, but it is highly likely that this may actually have saved the baby's life by permitting its chest and trunk to slip out more easily, allowing the baby to establish independent respiration.

With good care and attention the clavicle quickly healed and the injury didn't seem to have caused the baby any long-term effects. After taking this history from Rosemary, it was time to address her future birth. I said to her, 'So, this time round were you thinking of having a Caesarean section to avoid a similar situation?' She looked at me a little surprised and said, 'No, I wasn't.' I came back and said, 'It's just that quite often when something traumatic happens at one delivery a mother will often seriously consider a different route for delivery the next time so as to avoid a repeat episode. Rosemary, quick as a flash, came back to me with. 'No, no. To tell you truth, the way I look at it, it wasn't my clavicle!' Now, I know she didn't mean it the way it came out, though it did make me smile.

Was she being selfish? Or was she being sensible? There is absolutely no doubt it was the latter! Shoulder dystocia in a healthy pregnancy can be a frightening scenario for all concerned, but it is highly unlikely to recur in subsequent pregnancies especially if the staff at the delivery know that this has happened in a previous pregnancy and are well prepared.

Rosemary went on to have a straightforward pregnancy and this time the baby's shoulders followed the head spontaneously and did not require any well-practised but rarely used medical or midwifery interventions and manoeuvres.

Rosemary is a fine example of a woman who wants to make

choices and be in control of her pregnancy. It's a laudable and very acceptable stance, and should be encouraged by health professionals. However, there is another group of women, equally entitled to their view, who like having medical professionals around them who will take over much of the control and decision-making during labour. One woman explained it to me once by saying, 'Listen doctor, when I go to see my kid's teacher at school, she doesn't ask me how I want my child taught. She tells me how she is going to teach him. I want you to treat me in the same way.'

One can see a similar diversity of opinion when it comes to antenatal classes. Some women simply choose not to attend. I recall asking a young mother at my clinic whether she was attending these classes where she could find out about what to expect in labour and so forth, and her reply was 'No, I don't need to go to those classes.' I quickly glanced at her chart to confirm that this was indeed her first pregnancy. It was, so I said, 'But you haven't been in a labour ward since you were born! Don't you think it would be good to know what to expect?' Her reply summed up the thinking of many young mums today, and I loved it. She said, and truly meant, 'I don't need to go to classes because I'm having an epidural. My friend told me that was the way to go.'

It's my hormones, doctor

As obstetricians and gynaecologists, we often enter the profession because of the emotions we experience the first time we are privileged to observe a birth. My own experience of this sent shivers up and down my spine and that wonderful reflex response to birth has endured throughout my professional life.

As my career has progressed, this feeling has only been matched by the huge joy I have felt as a gynaecologist when I have successfully helped to address complaints associated with the sometimes adverse effects of a patient's hormones. We all have sex hormones. In men they tend to be fairly steady on a day-to-day basis, as they are in women who are pregnant, breastfeeding or well past the menopause. However, they can be anything but steady in a woman in her fertile years who is not pregnant and who is not taking a combined hormonal preparation for birth control. Sometimes the hormonal milieu that occurs in women at this stage of life can cause problems that have been variously described as premenstrual tension, syndrome or dysphoric disorder. The condition is often characterised by physical and psychosomatic symptoms that include fluid retention, mood swings, irritability, abdominal swelling and breast engorgement with tenderness. Some of these symptoms are probably noted by most woman in their fertile years, but in around 3 per cent of women, the condition is regarded as significant and needs medical attention.

Most symptoms, at least initially, respond to healthy diet and lifestyle changes, but a few require medical intervention. Many more women in the resourced world seek attention for these hormonal problems than in in the under-resourced world. One reason why there are such huge differences in the numbers is that women in the under-resourced world do not menstruate as often as their Western counterparts. This is down to the fact that many Western woman are now able to exercise a great deal of choice about their reproductive lives.

It is only relatively recently that some women have had the choice whether they want to be incessantly pregnant, plus or minus the associated breastfeeding, throughout their reproductive years. Before this shift, many women were not able to make their own reproductive choices and their lives followed a fairly common pattern. The onset of menstruation in a young girl in her teens was followed, one or two years later, by the onset of ovulation and ensuing potential fertility. In many cultures, the onset of menstruation triggered the young girl being married to a member of the opposite sex, and pregnancy ensued.

When a baby was born it was breastfed, and this method of feeding led to a cessation of menstruation and ovulation for the period during which the baby was breastfed. Conception during this time is therefore unlikely to occur. If a woman breastfed for five years then it was possible for her to have a total of four or five children during her fertile years, with a gap of four to five years between each child. We know this because primates, who appear to be unbothered by social, religious, peer or cultural pressures, do indeed have families of this type and size if left totally to nature. Fertility decreases greatly when a woman reaches her forties, and just about all chances of a naturally occurring pregnancy disappear at the age of fifty when menstruation stops, the menopause begins and women prepare for an increasingly lengthy post-reproductive life of three or more decades. A woman fulfilling her apparently natural reproductive role in the traditional way that I have described will have a total of sixty to ninety periods throughout her life. This is still the pattern for women in much of the world.

This menstrual pattern has shifted radically for women in the contemporary resourced world. Here the age of the menopause has remained fairly static over the past century, but the age of the menarche has been getting lower and lower to the point where it is not unusual for a girl of nine or ten to experience the onset of her periods. This change is associated with the increasing external sensory stimulation of the higher centres of the brain by exposure to TV and other multimedia, better diet and the increased sexualisation of children. Interestingly much international work suggests that girls who live in an urban environment begin menstruating up to two years earlier than girls who live in a rural environment, and there is also a strong theory that increased exposure to light in the home and from the computer screen may stimulate the pineal gland, which then stops producing melatonin, and the consequences of this series of events releases the body to develop sexually. Only a few decades ago menstruation at the age of nine would have been regarded by a gynaecologist as a sign of precocious (abnormally early) puberty. Now it is taken as normal.

When menstruation starts later, at fifteen or sixteen years of age, with ovulation and fertility beginning two years later, a woman is much better equipped to decide when and with whom she should share that fertility. It is expecting a lot of a girl, who has started menstruating at nine or ten, to avoid intimacy and preganancy for at least a decade. Many manage to negotiate this difficult territory, but others do not, for a variety of sociological reasons. For doctors managing birth control and the consequences of its absence in this group of young teenagers, this shift presents a real challenge, though I have always found it useful to remember this maxim passed on to me by a very sensible family planning doctor: 'It is our responsibility as doctors to look after a young girl's body until such time as her mind catches up.'

Over the next decade or so after menstruation begins, a

young girl in the resourced world will have a continuous and, one might say, incessant succession of the menstrual episodes associated with ovulation and the allied hormonal changes. In the forty years between the onset of menstruation and the menopause, a woman will potentially be subject to occasional contraception, plus or minus the personal choice of prolonged virginity and chastity. On average a woman will have two children, and statistically she will not breastfeed them for long, if at all. It is entirely possible, indeed probable, that a woman from a developed country could have an average of four hundred and fifty periods in her lifetime. Quite a difference from sixty.

My long gynaecological career has brought me into contact with many women suffering from hormonal problems and treating them has led me to spend some time considering the following questions. Are incessant menstruation, ovulation, and the premenstrual state actually detrimental to some women's health? Is there a need to routinely menstruate and ovulate if pregnancy is not desired? Could it be more beneficial to suppress ovulation and menstruation – as nature does during pregnancy and lactation – when a woman is avoiding pregnancy?

In the main, gynaecologists tend to deal with hormonal problems that affect women either pre-menstrually or peri-menopausally. Unfortunately, women who have premenstrual problems are more prone to having a more difficult time at the menopause. During the normal menstrual cycle, nature makes a woman appear to be at her most receptive, perhaps her most attractive, and her most apparently fertile in the time up to and around the middle of the month, ten to fourteen days after menstruation starts, so that if a pregnancy is desired, then appropriate steps can be taken. If pregnancy does not occur by accident or design, nature itself isn't really that fussed on how the woman feels in the days prior to the next menstruation, when she sheds the now redundant lining of the womb.

I am totally supportive of every empowered woman who decides not to have children. But this massive change in lifestyle choice that has occurred for many women in the resourced world in the twentieth century has happened at such a speed that evolution just hasn't caught up as yet.

Penny's story makes the issues clear. Penny was a thirty-six-year-old working mother, who was trying to keep body, soul, family, marriage, relationships with colleagues and sanity together while a maelstrom of hormonal changes whipped through her body for anything from two to twenty days every month. At the age of fifteen, Penny's GP had very wisely prescribed the contraceptive pill, as her menstrual pattern was interfering with her ability to concentrate, to pass exams, play sport – to live a normal life. The pill has emancipated women by giving them birth control, but equally or more importantly it has given many women cycle control so as they can perform consistently, month in, month out.

At university Penny met Fred, the love of her life, and, following graduation, she settled down, stopped taking the pill and had the two children that she planned and desired. In her late twenties, following a mature conversation, or two or three, her husband had a vasectomy. Penny was delighted not to have to take the pill any longer, and she hoped that the few not-so-pleasant side effects that she had experienced over the years, such as occasional low libido and weight gain would disappear.

She told me she was delighted to stop the pill for two other reasons. First, she was fed up being the person in the relationship who took responsibility for birth control, and second, she was tired of the conflicting advice in the media, as to the benefits or otherwise of long-term pill usage.

By the time I saw Penny, some eight years after her husband's vasectomy, she was a menstrual and hormonal mess, who had ballooned to a size eighteen and had suffered a serious plunge in self-confidence. She had all the symptoms of a well-established premenstrual syndrome and those symptoms had been increasing in severity from the time she had stopped taking the pill. She told me, 'For ten days every month I know

I am terrible to live with, but I can't stop the words coming out of my mouth. While being this nightmare with my family, I can have a complete 180-degree turnaround when someone from outside is on the scene. Fred says that I'm all over them like a rash and as nice as ninepence.' Penny's family was shocked, hurt and not a little bit angry that this mostly caring wife and mother could be two different people at the same time. This kind of hormonal problem, often accompanied by this type of behaviour, is something I've heard from women on a weekly basis for over thirty-five years.

Penny related the rest of her history to me, and confided that the symptoms which she had attributed to the pill, such as weight gain and low libido, had worsened rather than improved.

There is a very understandable view taken by many women that the hormones in the female body are something that can be checked very easily by a blood test, and many women come to the hospital clinic with a letter from their GP that tells them that their hormones are normal. They are often very confused by this result, as it doesn't fit with how they are feeling in their bodies in general, and in their head in particular. Of course, a hormonal analysis with a 'normal' result simply confirms that the woman is still ovulating and is not menopausal. It does not confirm that a woman's behaviour, psyche or the physical symptoms of her response to her hormonal milieu are normal or acceptable to her.

It had been my privilege to deliver Penny's children all those years before, and I remembered her as a fit, attractive, motivated, confident woman. In front of me was an overweight, depressed-looking, round-shouldered, exhausted working mother.

I examined Penny, scanned her pelvis and found absolutely nothing wrong. Again, this was not greeted with any relief from Penny as she wanted me to find something that could be fixed to help her change the way she felt about life.

When addressing premenstrual syndrome issues, Penny had three options, and they would be the same for any women in this situation. First, she could learn to live with the symptoms and tackle them as far as possible with diet and exercise. This can be helpful for many. Second, we could treat the symptoms – such as breast tenderness, fluid retention, depression and so on – one by one, perhaps by the use of pharmaceutical agents and with or without alternative therapies. This approach is worthwhile in many cases. But by the time a woman attends a hospital for a consultation, she will probably already have tried alternative medicines, lifestyle changes and many drugs. And so – as I did with Penny – we often move straight to the third option, that of addressing the cause, which is the menstrual cycle itself.

The area of hormonal control of reproduction is centred in the pituitary gland which is to be found just behind the nose, at the base of the brain. This small organ produces all the chemical messengers that regulate hormones and ensures that they are released at the correct intervals and time. What we know as the 'hypothalamic pituitary ovarian axis' controls the release of hormones in a sequential manner with the best intentions at heart, so that there are regular ovulation opportunities for the woman that wishes to become pregnant. However, if left to occur on a monthly basis without a break, the relentless release of these hormones can sometimes lead to the equivalent of overheating of the whole system. Penny, it seemed to me, required a break from the incessant ovulation and incessant menstruation that she had experienced since she stopped taking the pill.

Apart from pregnancy, there are two ways of suppressing ovulation, and hence the cycle itself. We can expose the woman to the pill or other drugs that negate ovulation, or we can surgically remove the ovaries. When this procedure is performed, it is combined with the removal of the uterus (hysterectomy) as without ovaries, the uterus becomes a redundant organ.

Penny said that she was extremely reluctant to go back on the pill as she felt she had taken it for long enough and didn't like the idea of taking contraceptives she didn't require. Sometimes it's frustrating for those of us who work in this area that a combination of the two hormones, oestrogen and progesterone, is always described as the contraceptive pill because its uses are way beyond simply those of contraception. Women are constantly being harangued by the media about the effects of the pill: sometimes good, sometimes bad, and often conflicting advice can be offered in the same edition of a magazine. So, when a woman who has no need for its contraceptive properties is offered the drug to address another gynaecological complaint, there is frequently bewilderment at the advice. Penny just did not want to countenance taking the pill again, even though, for example, women who take HRT (hormone replacement therapy) are taking the same drugs that constitute the pill, but in smaller doses.

I suggested to Penny that we should give her the planned break from incessant ovulation and menstruation by exposing her to a very clever and powerful drug which mimics or blocks output from the pituitary 'control tower' altogether for a month at a time. Powerful drugs have powerful side effects, but it is my experience that women who are relieved of their premenstrual symptoms, even for a short while, are so delighted to feel better in themselves and to have a definite diagnosis that they can live with many of the side effects of the drugs.

I prescribed the drug for six months and during this time Penny had no periods and was without a cycle for the first time in almost a decade. I saw her again at the conclusion of her treatment and she walked into my consulting rooms looking like a new woman. Yes, she had experienced some side effects, as the therapy produces the symptoms of an instant menopause, but she said: 'Wow, where has this drug been all my life? Why have I had to put up with this? I really thought I was going mad. My kids were fed up with me and I think hated me, and my husband was staying well out of the way Now I have time to re-establish a great relationship with my children, and my husband and I are having a ball. I haven't addressed the weight gain yet, but whereas I used to look in the mirror and think, "Gosh you're fat!" now I look in the mirror and say, "Gosh I must go out and buy some new clothes that flatter the bigger me".'

I will never forget Penny saying that, as it proved that she didn't want to be someone else – she wanted to be herself, but happy and confident. Of course that wasn't the end of the story, but at least Penny knew there was an answer to the way she had been feeling and that she was on the road to having a much better life.

In fairness though, my choice of this particular story is a bit like putting your holiday photos on Facebook. You only post the good ones. Not all clinical problems can be addressed so successfully, but when they can, the result is life-changing for the woman. When I started my work in this field, gynaecology was seen very much as a surgical speciality. There wasn't much else to offer a woman with unacceptably heavy periods or the occasional functional problems, such as urinary and faecal incontinence, associated with childbirth. Nowadays, however, much of our work can be carried out in the office setting. Major surgery is now seen as a last resort. Pharmaceutical agents, which allow us to mimic nature, are available and allow us to address the damage to everyday living that incessant ovulation and menstruation can cause.

A tiny miracle

Looking after maternity patients is mostly a joy and always a privilege. There is, however, rarely time to find out very much about the woman behind the mother. The focus is on the clinical course of the pregnancy, the baby and its birth. Meeting the same patient in a gynaecological environment, however, often provides the time and the opportunity to find out a little about the woman's life and her past. When a gynaecologist meets a patient for the first time, there is a need to find out a bit about the woman's social, medical, surgical and obstetrical background in order to understand and treat her effectively. Factors such as the patient's age – any woman between fifteen and forty-five is often either pregnant or doing their best not to be in that condition – or the number of children already at home will also be part of the picture as well as the details of the woman's current gynaecological problem.

Recently I met Maisie, a very bright and bubbly eighty-two-year-old woman. Having introduced myself, I started to take a history. Maisie told me in a very matter-of-fact manner that she had two sons and that she had also experienced three miscarriages. With such a history and particularly in women of this age group, I often find that it is useful to enquire about the miscarriages – pregnancy loss in previous decades was often considered part of life, and there was little or no counselling available or offered. Very frequently older women will noticeably catch their breath when they mention that they lost a baby and it is not unusual for their eyes to well up with tears as they remember the circumstances involved. Often grief and loss have been buried in the past, along with the baby, and I find that a little bit of gentle prompting can be extremely helpful for everyone.

Times were hard after the First World War. Women tended to have more children than they do now and most women went into pregnancy in the knowledge that everything wouldn't necessarily work out well. Miscarriage, defined at that time as the loss of the baby at less than twenty-eight weeks gestation, was often dealt with in a very matter-of-fact way. Babies were often stillborn and no one was considered to blame. The prevalent attitude was: these things happen. Even when the baby was born alive, cot death could occur in the best-regulated households in the early months and the loss of a young baby from vomiting and diarrhoea, pneumonia, whooping cough or other infection was common. Parents' expectations of their children's life expectancy were much lower than they are today. Thankfully, many of the problems frequently observed by my former colleagues in the 1950s and 1960s have now been addressed, though some do remain.

I commented to Maisie that she appeared very pragmatic and sensible about her three miscarriages. She agreed and said, 'I believe, doctor, that if you have a healthy pregnancy, then you'll have a healthy baby, although I must say I did defy the odds myself.' I asked her to expand.

'Well, as you can see from my chart, doctor, I was born on 24 December 1929. I was my mother's third baby. I have an older brother and sister. My mother Rosalind was twenty-three weeks pregnant and had been charging around trying to get things organised for Christmas when she started having labour pains. My father was dispatched round to the GP's surgery to try and contact the local doctor and returned with the message that there wasn't an awful lot he could do to help at that stage of pregnancy, but that he would pop in later. Dad then called to the house of the local midwife and left a message with her husband to ask her to pop in to see my mum.

'Mum apparently carried on wrapping presents and stuffing the turkey until about four o'clock in the afternoon when the midwife called. She examined my mum and found that I was on my way. My mum, who was as practical as I am, was hoping that her miscarriage would be sorted out before the Christmas dinner needed to be cooked and served the next day.

'The midwife, however, stayed with mum and I popped out within the next hour or so, still within my own little fish bowl created by the bag of membranes around me, which were still intact. Mum says it was just as though I was swimming around in a mini swimming pool.

'Needless to say, no one had any hope for my survival. There was certainly no ambulance called, and intensive care units hadn't been invented! The midwife opened the bag of membranes and set me on a warm towel. Mum continued to have a very practical attitude and apparently held my hand for a while and no doubt said her goodbyes.

'As the midwife tidied up her bits and pieces, my dad came into the bedroom and, having checked that everything was okay with my mum, went over, looked at me on the towel and just apparently kept staring. The midwife apparently then said, "'There you are, Mr Thompson, it just wasn't meant to be. Still, it's good that you were around today and you were able to come and fetch me to help. Rosalind is doing well here and there doesn't seem to be anything else wrong." Dad then came over to look at me again, pulled open the blanket and said, "'But she's still alive." The midwife said, "Yes, she is at present but I wouldn't expect her to last more than half an hour."

'Dad was a very gentle man, although he worked very much in a man's world as he was a welder in the Belfast shipyards. I remember him as being very practical all my life. Apparently he went downstairs and got a shoebox, lined it with cotton wool and laid me down inside it. He told me years later that he could nearly see through me and that my eyes were fused but that my wee chest continued to move up and down very constantly and regularly.

'Olive oil was used regularly as a home remedy and was to be found in every house in the 1920s and he poured olive oil over me to keep the heat in and then set me down, in the box, beside the range in the kitchen, probably hoping that I would pass away very gently. I suppose he was caring for me in much the same way that a young child would tend for an injured bird. He said that he had a funny wee feeling about me. When he went back after an hour he expected me to be gone, but there I was breathing away. He and mum decided they would have to give me a name, so I became Maisie. On Christmas morning when he woke up, he was amazed to find that I was still hanging in there.

'Even though it was over eighty years ago, everyone understood the simple basics of life. Nourishment and warmth should be offered at the start of life and at its end. You will love this part of the story doctor, as I see you are writing with a Parker pen. On Christmas morning my mother gave my father a Parker pen as a present and dad immediately went to the kitchen and instead of filling it with ink, he filled it with milk from the top of the bottle. He dropped a little into my mouth, much as one would feed a little sparrow that had fallen out of its nest. Lo and behold, every time he came back to me, there I was breathing away and with my mouth open and looking for more milk. I became the talk of the town around Willowfield in east Belfast.

'After Christmas other members of the family and even dad's workmates popped in and asked to have a look at me. Eventually, I was the talk of the shipyard as well! Of course everyone thought that dad was mad and that he was wasting his time, but apparently I just kept thriving on this cow's milk. He never once lifted me out of the box but simply kept pouring olive oil over me as I lay on my cotton wool bed. Finally, I started piddling and pooing and he did nothing more dramatic than change the cotton wool at the lower end.

'Although Mum and my sister were both involved, it seems that Dad was the key man and, although he kept going to work, he spent the rest of his time worrying about me and asking everyone he met what he should do next. It seems I sailed through everything and became a little bit more vigorous day by day.

'In the New Year, Dad went to the GP and discussed my prognosis. The GP was both intrigued and flabbergasted at my progress and suggested the following mixture for nutrition: fresh minced liver, the juice of an Outspan orange, five spoonfuls of Five Star Brandy, all mixed up in cow's milk. This is what I was fed on through the Parker pen, until I could take a bottle. Soon my eyes opened and my skin became normal looking. Clothes had to be found for me, but none existed that were small enough in the shops and so I was dressed in my sister's dolls clothing throughout the first month of my life.

'Finally, I was able to leave my shoebox beside the range, and was weaned off the diet of brandy and orange juice. I was moved to a crib beside mum's bed and started to follow the same diet as my brother and sister. Apparently I never looked back.

'When I did go to school, I turned out to be pretty bright and indeed I was third in the United Kingdom in mental arithmetic exams. I have entered many local and national quizzes all my life and have won most of them. Of course, things weren't great for girls in the 1940s and I had to leave school at fourteen years of age. However, I was an avid reader, they couldn't stop me doing that! I ended up being the PA to the head of a big corporation in Belfast until such times as I got married, when of course I was sacked. I then fulfilled the role that had been mapped out for women in those days. I ran the home and had my own two children. So there you are, doctor, what do you think of that?'

I was almost speechless and couldn't believe that the incredibly fit-looking octogenarian sitting in front of me had been born weighing less than a pound (approximately 400g) and had gone through life with practically no medical problems. Hope, indeed, does spring eternal and where there is life, there is hope. Maisie's dad had hope, and Maisie proved that it's more important *how* you are born and cared for, than *when* you appear in this world.

I treated Maisie's relatively minor gynaecological problem and she was ready to be on her way. She did, however, allow me to take a picture of her, which I keep to this day. She also gave me permission to write about her and, as one of the founders and current president of TinyLife, the premature baby charity in Northern Ireland, I have used that story often to bring hope to parents of premature babies.* As Maisie was about to leave the room, she turned around and said, 'Oh, and another thing, doctor, you will know yourself that it was pretty unusual to be born inside your own membranes and it is considered a sign of luck for us here in Ireland. Well, wait till you hear, the midwife took the membranes and let them dry out and sold them to a ship's captain for fifty pounds. He kept them in his wallet all his life to bring him good luck when he was at sea. From what I hear, it worked rightly.'

It is tempting to believe that nature always gets it right and that all pregnancies that miscarry are just nature sorting things out. That is probably correct, nine times out of ten, but every so often there are opportunities to stop nature in its tracks.

Ethicists, politicians and lawyers are probably more concerned about gestational time landmarks during the pregnancy cycle than we medics are – we see the mother and her pregnancy as a clinical continuum. However, for very good reasons,

---

* In 1988 Garth McClure, a good friend and paediatric colleague, and I set up a charity in Northern Ireland to help address the awful loss of babies born prematurely. It is a credit to the many researchers, the Department of Health in Northern Ireland who fund the intensive care units, and healthcare providers that death from prematurity after twenty-four weeks rarely occurs in Northern Ireland now. This means that the TinyLife charity can now focus on supporting parents to care for their babies when they are discharged from hospital, rather than simply having survival as an end point.

there is much discussion at many levels of society as to when conception actually occurs; at what point life begins; when a pregnancy is viable; when a pregnancy loss is considered to be a birth or a miscarriage; and what the expected date of delivery is. As doctors, though, we do not spend our lives running around with a calculator to gauge what our attitude should be to a woman at any particular time in her pregnancy. If a woman has a problem, it is dealt with on the basis of her clinical need, rather than any other parameter.

A mother's life is sacred and I am delighted that in my lifetime I have seen a huge change in attitude in the developed world so that now, at last, a mother's mental health is considered to have the same importance as her physical state. This change in attitude is increasingly being reflected by the deliberations and decisions of politicians and lawmakers. For us on the ground though, it is something we have known for as long as I can remember. One can often be in consultation with a woman who is physically extremely healthy but is a mental wreck, and similarly, and perhaps ironically, we often see women who are physically weak but are mentally strong and resilient. As doctors, we now spend our time assessing and trying to improve health in both areas.

The Law Lords, responding to the introduction of the morning-after pill, have ruled on when conception occurs. Does it occur when the sperm enters the egg or does it occur when the fertilised egg embeds into the uterus? The Law Lords have deemed that the first event is simply physiological, whereas the second event, when the fertilised egg becomes attached to the mother by embedding into the uterus, is designated as conception. This is of major legal importance as any actions taken to prevent implantation of a fertilised egg are now classified as contraception rather than abortion.

Much of our time as obstetricians is spent trying to prevent miscarriages and premature births. Any medical decision, therefore, to encourage the womb to expel its contents is never taken lightly and is always made either with the aim of providing the parents with the best clinical option based on the mother's physical and mental needs or because the fetus must be delivered before it dies. As obstetricians, we must observe the law and take cognisance of the point in the gestational spectrum that a problem occurs, but the problem itself does not change because of the date on the Gregorian calendar.

One of the most difficult questions to address is fetal viability – identifying the point at which the fetus can survive outside the womb – and, related to this, the question of whether induction of labour at a stage when the baby could not survive outside the womb, constitutes abortion. Trying to legislate around such issues is a subject of ongoing passionate debate from all sides. When I qualified in 1973, the legal definition of fetal viability was twenty-eight weeks gestation. It is now twenty-four weeks. In the 1920s Maisie defied the odds and the medics' expectations, but not her father's hopes, when she was born and survived at twenty-three weeks. By the legal definitions of the time, she spent the first five weeks of her life as a 'miscarriage', but by general consensus of all she was, and is, a miracle.

Consequences

Good nursing can sometimes be all a patient needs to return to good health. The early NHS provided this in spades. Add to this appropriate pharmaceutical agents and surgical interventions that are evidence-based, and we have a recipe for taking on nature when she has decided that we are no longer 'fit for purpose'.

Drugs, whether based on naturally occurring flora or fauna, or concocted in the laboratory, are potentially very powerful and often produce good effects and/or serious side effects. Either way, they have consequences. When contemplating the prescription of drugs for pregnant women, such considerations must be taken even more seriously. It may come as a surprise that the prescribing bible, the *British National Formulary*, is very light on advice on what to use for pregnant women and children, never mind for the fetus at its various stages of development. Ethical committees are understandably reluctant to support studies on children, and so fairly simple logical approaches, based on adult studies that then take into account the child's weight, tend to be used when prescribing drugs in this group.

'No drugs at all' is a worthy and noble stance to take in pregnancy … if only life was so simple. In early pregnancy mothers may have myriad complaints, all associated with the fine-tuning of their bodies being upset by the hormone push of the developing embryo and its placenta. Amongst the most common of complaints is morning sickness, which produces nausea that is similar to travel sickness in general, and seasickness in particular. Morning sickness can be anything from a few symptoms every morning to the full-blown condition, *hyperemesis gravidarum*, when the mother can literally keep nothing down and can quickly become very ill indeed. Before there were any treatments for this condition, some women had to have their pregnancies terminated to prevent their untimely death. Charlotte Brontë, for example, is generally thought to have died of the condition. Even if death was avoided, the associated dehydration and vitamin deficiencies could lead to a condition known as 'Wernicke's encephalopathy', which causes serious loss of coordination as well as confusion and delirium. So, when pharmaceutical companies approached the medical fraternity in the middle of the last century with thalidomide – a new drug that really worked for morning sickness – there was a strong impetus to get it to patients as quickly as possible.

When thalidomide came onto the market, doctors and midwives at last felt they had something effective to recommend to women with morning sickness. After some time the catastrophic side effects on the developing embryo were recognised worldwide. The drug was withdrawn from use for morning sickness and the rest is tragic history. A key consequence of the thalidomide story was a major reassessment by the medical fraternity, worldwide, of the harmful effects of drugs on the developing embryo and fetus, and a recognition that never again should a drug be recommended before it had undergone rigorous testing. In the twenty-first century the medical profession is much more knowledgeable about what drugs cross over to the fetus, in what quantities, and their potential effects and side effects. It's not all about avoiding the fetus being affected, though. Many fetuses can be intentionally treated through drugs administered to the mother. For example, over the last thirty years, the administration of fairly low-dose steroids to the mother, antenatally, at the correct time and in the correct manner, has had a hugely positive effect on reducing the incidence of respiratory distress in the premature newborn.

Sir Graham (Mont) Liggins was the eminent Australian scientist, physiologist and researcher who cracked the relationship – and the ensuing therapeutic advantages – between the administration of steroids to mothers and the lessening of problems of respiration for the prematurely born infant. In the 1970s, he was one of a team of doctors studying the physiology behind the onset of labour. We still don't really know what brings on labour in women but many of the pieces of the jigsaw are slowly falling into place. When Liggins was carrying out his groundbreaking work, however, the picture was very far from complete. The rationale for his investigations was that if scientists could work out the sequence of events that caused the onset of labour in normal circumstances, they would have a much better chance of learning how to prevent that very labour when it occurred prematurely in abnormal ones.

Countless millions of babies die every year worldwide because, often for no apparent reason, the mother's womb starts contracting too early and the baby is born prematurely. At the time Liggins was studying this problem, there was a general consensus that steroids played some part in the triggering process of the initiation of labour. In order to aid their investigations, Liggins and his team did a lot of work in very sophisticated laboratories with sheep. Many animals have their own particular mechanism for giving birth, but sheep appear to have some similar neurophysiological pathways to humans when it comes to labour onset. Unlike humans, for whom the term of a pregnancy can be anything from thirty-seven to forty-two weeks, sheep have an incredibly accurate gestation period of 147 days and only have a twenty-four- to forty-eight-hour window in which they give birth.

Liggins and his team administered quite large doses of steroids to the pregnant ewe in the hope of triggering premature labour at or around the 120-day mark, and indeed were successful. They were intrigued to note that the newborn lambs had very few of the expected respiratory problems. Usually, premature sheep, or premature humans for that matter, have a lack of the fluid in their lungs that lowers surface tension. This lack means that when the little lung sacs collapse as the sheep, or baby, breathes out, they can't expand easily again when the sheep, or baby, tries to inhale. The missing fluid is known as surfactant, or surface active material, and when high-quality surfactant is present in appropriate amounts, the lungs can expand and contract at will, without too much effort or distress.

Liggins put forward the theory that the steroids must have not only triggered the onset of labour, but also rapidly stimulated the maturation of the fetal lungs. In addition, more refined work thereafter suggested that fairly small doses of the same drug administered to the mother could give the same positive benefit to the fetal lungs but without stimulating the birth process. Administering low-dose steroids to mothers at risk of premature birth is now accepted worldwide, and millions of babies are saved needless distress and death as a result of these research findings.

However in the twilight of my obstetric career, I do often ponder the effects, good and maybe not so good, of the treatments and therapeutic interventions we have offered over the years. During my time working in Canada, where I was seconded in 1976 just two years into my career pathway in obstetrics and gynaecology, I worked with a great team of doctors. One of the team, who had come to Canada from Scotland, still had nightmares at the thought of how many women for whom, with the best of intentions, he had prescribed thalidomide in the 1960s to help with crippling morning sickness. Thalidomide is still used to this day, often following transplant surgery, because of its anti-rejection properties.

In the 1970s and 80s, a vast number of pregnant women throughout the developed world were treated very readily and quite heavily with large amounts of Valium (a brand of diazepam). This was no doubt correctly prescribed for its anti-anxiety properties. The finding of a couple of maternal elevated blood pressure measurements was enough to initiate treatment with Valium as the dangers of untreated hypertension can be very severe for the mother and her fetus. However one can only speculate on the possible unintentional effects, if any, the drug had on the neurobehavioural development of the fetus in the last months of pregnancy. Might it be a contributory factor to drug use/abuse later in life? Could mothers who had been exposed to mind-affecting drugs in pregnancy give birth to babies who were more likely to be prone to addiction in later life? Certainly today my paediatric colleagues are frequently called upon to deal with the cold turkey experienced by the newborn with a drug-addicted mother. To every action there is an equal and opposite reaction, as Newton surmised some time ago.

In the 1960s, 70s and 80s, women with a history of recurrent miscarriage were frequently given weekly injections of the female hormone progesterone to help prevent them from miscarrying next time round. Evidence-based medicine now suggests that, while the logic appeared sound, the treatment was probably not required for many of the pregnancies for which it was prescribed. One is left again surmising what possible long-term effect, if any, this sex hormone could have had on a developing fetus of either gender.

There is, though, a hugely understandable stance taken by all concerned in the care of women who have endured miscarriages – that it is necessary to 'do something'. This 'something' is often adding a pharmaceutical agent or performing a surgical procedure that will somehow bamboozle nature into holding on to the pregnancy that is so yearned for by the parents. The feelings of loss and inadequacy experienced by a woman who miscarries a desired baby will make parents search the world for a treatment that will enable them to have a child, and drives the rest of us to exhaust all the means at our disposal to find a solution. But we have a big responsibility only to prescribe and administer therapies that truly work.

In my professional life I have witnessed many agents and operations being used to help overcome the threat of miscarriage but nature is usually a fair, if ruthless, taskmaster in this area. Give her good materials and she rarely makes a mistake. The maxim, 'before doing any good, make sure you do no harm' is worth keeping at the forefront of your mind when prescribing during pregnancy.

When a woman goes into labour, the pain caused by the contractions cause her to produce and release her own morphine-like endorphins which provide some measure of relief from the discomfort she may be experiencing. Normally, though, endorphins are released in a controlled way, by starting or stopping exercise, for example. During labour, however, the release of endorphins cannot be so adjusted. Those that are released cross the placenta to the fetus and no doubt help provide relief for any discomfort the fetus may experience when it is passing through the pelvis, and especially, perhaps, when an assisted delivery is being performed with the use of vacuum or forceps. Therefore it seems logical that the maternally supplied endorphins have a protective effect on the fetus. Similarly, when midwives and doctors administer pain relief in the form of pethidine (Demerol) to the mother, some of that drug is of course transferred to the fetal circulation, thus providing the fetus with similar 'pain relief'. But let's consider what happens to the fetus when a mother has an epidural. She is pain free, no endorphins are being released, and the fetus is as compos mentis as its mother but, it could be argued, it is now deficient of naturally occurring maternal endorphins during any subsequent assisted delivery.

Having observed the outcome of labours during both the heavily-sedated-mother era and the more contemporary epidural one, the latter appears to be much superior for mum and baby.

One problem, though, is that sometimes an epidural doesn't work too well, or only works on one side. For that particular mother, that scenario is probably worse than not having an epidural at all. For when the mother does not have an epidural, her carers will prescribe other methods of pain relief or therapies but when the epidural is in place but not working, they tend not to treat or address the non-working segment as much as they should or could.

Epidurals sometimes work extra well and their effects can be felt much higher up the body than intended. I once cared for a mother whose epidural effects went so high that she couldn't move her lower jaw! The anaesthetist was quite concerned until the unintended effects wore off. The same mother, however, came back two years later for another baby and said to me, 'Prof, remember that epidural I had the last time – it went right up to my neck?' I reassured her that it was probably a one-off experience, but she interrupted me and said, 'Oh no, please, I would like one exactly the same as that again. It was magic!' Just goes to show.

Wiped out

While there have been no major changes in women or the process of pregnancy in the last centuries, there certainly have been major changes in the way in which we address problems when things don't go quite as they should during birth. Much learning for doctors nowadays relies, quite correctly, on the use of simulation exercises, the frequent practice of skills and drills, and adherence to evidence-based guidelines. As far as they go, these are all extremely helpful methods, but they can't be relied upon to prepare the obstetrician for all the real-life problems he/she may encounter. Much of my training was spent sitting in labour wards and doctor's messes, swapping clinical scenarios and describing solutions to clinical problems.

Ken Houston, a now retired consultant in the Jubilee Maternity Hospital, was one of those men who had dedicated his professional life to the care of women and over his forty-plus years in medicine, he pretty much saw it all. Ken was a junior doctor at the Jubilee in the late 1950s and he told me a story that demonstrated just how unpredictable a working shift could be.

He was on duty one night with his colleague, George Wilton, and they were both sitting having coffee in the sister's office in the labour ward. They were just commenting on how quiet a night it had been, when sister came in to say that there was a problem with Audrey Bell in Room 3 in the labour ward.

Mrs Bell was thirty-nine years old and had been married

for twenty years. She was pregnant with her first child. Her labour, so far, had been very long and she was exhausted. Mrs Bell was in the second stage of labour. In the first stage of labour the womb muscle contracts and retracts regularly to such a point that the cervix, which lies at the top of the birth canal, but the bottom of the womb, completely opens up (usually to 10cm) and allows the baby to descend and be born. Once the baby starts to descend, aided by the mother actively pushing, we are entering the second stage of labour, which finishes once the baby is delivered. The third stage of labour is considered to be complete when the placenta is delivered. Nature of course sees the whole thing as a continuum, which it is most times.

Mrs Bell had been in the second stage of labour and had pushing for an hour or more but seemed to have stopped making progress. Ken went to check on the situation. It was midnight and Ken was hoping that he could do a quick lift-out with forceps and then get to bed to try to grab an hour's sleep before he was required somewhere else in the hospital.

Examination of Mrs Bell, however, revealed that the baby's head was stuck in what we call the 'deep transverse arrest' position, where the baby's head is deep in the pelvis, but won't spontaneously turn to the side as it rotates down and through the birth canal, as it's meant to do in normal labour, since everything is just a bit too tight. In normal labour, the head enters the pelvis in a transverse position, with the baby's head to the side facing the mother's left or right hip. During the labour process the head usually corkscrews 90 degrees and the baby appears externally with the back of its head facing upwards and its face pointing downwards. Sometimes, the head just won't rotate and it stays in the transverse position. Particularly when a woman has had children before, we can help by manually rotating the baby's head round, or augment nature's contractions with drugs. Failing that, we either use instruments to deliver the baby or carry out a Caesarean section, depending on our estimation of the size of the baby, the size of the pelvis and our assessment of the amount of power that has been used.

Having examined Mrs Bell, Ken decided that her pelvis seemed adequate. Intravenous Oxytocin had not yet been invented and therefore there was no possibility of increasing the power. The baby had managed to get itself down to the point where its head could be said to be engaged, but it could rotate and descend no further. In this situation, Ken turned to the use of forceps invented by a Swedish obstetrician called Kjelland. They had two major differences from routine forceps. Their particular positive features were that they could be applied to the baby's head in the deep transverse position, and that the head could be rotated, theoretically, without damaging the mother or the baby. This was not always the case in practice, and although they have saved lives on many occasions, their use has decreased in the developed world as Caesarean sections became safer, and became the preferred way to address this problem.

Ken went in to see George and said, 'George, this woman needs a Kjelland's forceps, so one of us needs to provide the anaesthetic and one the forceps.' George, who eventually became an anaesthetist, said he would do the upper end if Ken would do the lower end. Anaesthesia in 1958 was not what it is today, and the option of a spinal anaesthetic where the patient is awake and conscious, but pain free, was not available. Instead, George had to administer chloroform via a face mask that provided the amount of anaesthetic required to reduce the consciousness of the patient and her response to pain.

The procedure started off well enough. Ken, using the full range of his skills, applied the forceps appropriately, and George was happy with how the anaesthesia was working. Ken did get the baby's head rotated, but there was little sign of it appearing through the traditional route. In the absence of the hoped-for outcome, Ken reported to George and the assembled midwifery staff that they would be best to resort to Caesarean section. It was certainly unusual to have to do a Caesarean section in these circumstances, but when the head won't come easily, there really is no other option.

Ken removed the forceps and went to prepare himself to perform a Caesarean section. Bikini incisions were something that came in the early 1970s and so the old-fashioned straight-up-and-down midline scar from Mrs Bell's umbilicus downwards was completed. As he made the incision, Ken noticed that the blood that appeared was not the bright pink type we all hopefully have pumping round our veins and arteries, but was a worryingly dark colour. George concurred, and a further check confirmed to them both that Mrs Bell had just experienced a cardiac arrest. Again, cardiac arrest teams had not been invented, and cardiac massage was amazingly and frequently successfully performed directly by manual massage of the heart rather than external compression. So Ken, using the same scalpel that he had used to incise Mrs Bell's abdomen, correctly made a small incision below her left breast in order to allow his hand to gain access to her heart and thereby pump it manually. However, having made the incision, he was just about to insert his hand when he realised that her life blood was pink again, and indeed, simultaneously, George confirmed that Mrs Bell's heart had spontaneously restarted. Both doctors then realised that their other patient, the baby, could also have been deprived of oxygen for that period of time and needed urgent delivery. Mind you, babies can come through an awful lot without suffering long-term damage. For pretty complicated but fascinatingly unique physiological reasons, adults can suffer brain damage after only four minutes of total oxygen deprivation, whereas a fetus would need up to twenty minutes of similar deprivation to cause the same injury. Also, when a mother has a cardiac arrest, the baby certainly doesn't follow suit, and can continue to pump blood around its brain from the reserves of blood in the placenta.

Ken wisely abandoned the idea of doing a Caesarean section and immediately went down to where the process had started. Time was of the essence. At least the baby's head was rotated to the right direction. He put on the standard forceps this time, and provided the required traction to effect the birth of the baby – who cried immediately and gave momentary delight to the whole team.

With the baby out and crying and everyone's heart now pumping normally, Ken proceeded to sew up Mrs Bell's three wounds: the one that he had to make in the birth canal (episiotomy) in order to effect a forceps delivery; the one for the Caesarean section that never happened; and the one below her left breast. George allowed Mrs Bell to come round from her anaesthetic and he and Ken were both delighted when she coughed and spluttered, and within a short while she was able to open an eye and smile at her beautiful baby. There would be plenty of time to tell her the whole saga later, and explain to her why she was perhaps a little sore in at least three areas. Now was the time for positive news only.

Ken and George were shattered. It was five o'clock in the morning. They sat in sister's office eating cheese on toast, and smoked their way through their own cigarettes and then everybody else's. The light was beginning to come up over Belfast when Ken suddenly realised that they hadn't informed the husband of the outcome of the near-perilous night.

Ken went downstairs to the waiting room, which was in the basement of the Jubilee, and there they found Mr Bell, who had been sitting with other fathers in the fairly spartan room. Mr Bell stood up as soon as Ken, who was still in shock himself, walked into the room. Ken informed him that he was the father of a healthy baby boy. Mr Bell was obviously thrilled and grateful for the news, but then Ken blurted out that it had been a close shave for both the baby and the mother. Ken himself admits that it was probably a bit more detail than was necessary. Mr Bell had seen some sights in his time but he had never been in a hospital before and had been waiting for twenty years for his son to arrive. It was all too much for him and he fainted in front of Ken, crashing to the floor and banging his head on the terrazzo floor. Blood started pouring from a big gash above his eye and Ken had another emergency on his hands. Ken and other fathers in the room got Mr Bell onto a trolley and, with their help, Ken immediately took him to the hospital's casualty department, where he received the necessary sutures from the casualty officer on duty.

With Mr Bell's injury dealt with, Ken went back to check on Mrs Bell and baby Bell. Both were ridiculously and delightfully well. It was now 8.30 a.m. and Ken and George were, at last, due to go off-duty in thirty minutes.

They went over to the doctor's mess and sat down at the breakfast table. Neither of them could think of anything to say. At five minutes to nine George went upstairs and came down with a bottle of Black Bush whiskey. He poured them both a drink. They threw the first couple back very quickly and then set themselves down to some serious consumption over a rather prolonged period of time.

As Ken put it to me all those years later, 'we didn't need to say too much to each other, as we just sat there thinking how – in one eight-hour period, with all the efforts of nature plus the two of us – we nearly wiped out a whole family in one fell swoop.'

The women of the Shankill

The Mater Infirmorum Hospital on the Crumlin Road in Belfast reflected, in many ways, the intricacies and oddities of Northern Ireland life in the twentieth century. Although it isn't the case now, back in the 1970s the Mater was perceived as having Catholic medical staff even though the hospital tended to look after the Protestant patients of the Shankill Road, while the Royal Victoria Hospital, less than a mile away, was perceived as having Protestant consultants but tended to look after the Catholic people of the Falls Road who lived in the immediate area.

I worked in both hospitals during my training. A central committee appointed trainees in obstetrics and gynaecology to the various units throughout Northern Ireland. I was appointed to the Mater Hospital as registrar on 1 August 1977, my first such appointment. There were two consultants in the Mater Hospital at that time, Joe Verzin and Rory Casement. The former was a papal knight who gained this honour as a result of his sterling international work in encouraging the abandonment of Female Genital Mutilation (FGM) in certain parts of Africa. He was well known for starting every lecture to a new group of nurses and midwives with the statement, 'I am an obstetrician and gynaecologist and a Roman Catholic, but I am primarily a Roman Catholic.' He was diligent and industrious in his care of the women he treated throughout his working life.

Rory Casement was also a Roman Catholic but often told me that his Catholicism was similar to an old but much-loved, well worn and comfortable coat that you kept hanging on the nail on the back of the kitchen door – it was always there to put on in times of hardship to give you warmth and protection. Rory was, along with Harith Lamki, Ken Houston and Buster Holland, one of the consultants who had a profound effect on my progress in obstetrics and gynaecology.

In the fullness of time, Rory told me that when I was appointed to the Mater, he was informed by the appointment committee that he should 'watch me carefully'. About a month after I joined the Mater, he invited me into his office for a chat and a review of my progress – I think management now call it an appraisal! He made it very clear that he wanted me to be myself, so that he could see what some members, or one member in particular of said committee, was concerned about. Many years afterwards Rory told me that one member, who believed I could be a bit anti-establishment in my behaviour, had suggested that I had only received such a glowing reference from a certain paediatrician because of my religion! Rory apparently said nothing at the interview, but apparently chuckled to himself as he knew that I did NOT practise the same faith as the paediatrician! Ah, the advantages of having a name that confuses the interested observer. Names were of huge importance in Northern Ireland and, combined with information of what school one attended, were often enough often to indicate a person's religious affiliation. I once asked a colleague why he and his wife named their third child Concepta, to which he mischievously replied, 'That's to save them asking the second question!'

To some extent, I can see how I was perceived as anti-establishment. I had been an active member of the local Junior Doctors' Committee that had successfully taken on Barbara Castle to get doctors paid for the work they did beyond fifty hours per week. At that time, doctors regularly worked 120 hours per week. I reassured Rory that I was being myself and we continued to work together happily for a whole year.

Rory treated all women with total and equal respect. There are many adjectives I could use to describe him: he was strong, polite, generous in nature, had a wicked sense of humour, was a genius in some ways, compassionate, warm, tolerant and brave. I saw examples of all of these qualities on many occasions. Joe Verzin, on the other hand, was very precise and careful with his work and although I respected him as much as other colleagues I worked with during my professional life, I didn't feel inspired or nurtured by him or most of the others in the way I did with Rory.

I was the only obstetric registrar in the Mater Hospital that year, and covered the hospital from home, seven miles away, every night of the week and every weekend of that year, except Tuesday nights and one weekend per month. Long hours – but the huge positive was that you certainly got to know the patients well. Continuity of care – such a massive problem for the NHS today, constrained as it is by the European Working Time Directive – was never an issue. I think there were around eight hundred deliveries per year at the Mater at that time, and you got to know everyone, patients and staff, individually, so that when you were phoned up at night by the house officer, he didn't say 'I have a twenty-five-year-old para 2 [short for 'parity', a technical term that refers to the number of times a woman has given birth to a baby] at thirty-nine weeks who has a problem', but rather, 'Roberta Jones has come in yet again!'

Hospital management in the 1970s was still carried out on a day-to-day basis by doctors and midwives working together via various committees. As registrar, I was invited along to the hospital meetings on a regular basis. Indeed we were such a small medical team that even house officers were invited along to make up the numbers and give the meetings an air of importance and respectability! My strong sense then was that management bodies were working for the good of the medical profession as a whole and to maximise outcomes for patients. Now, at the conclusion of my career, I feel strongly that something vital has been lost at the management level and that bodies in the UK are now acting primarily to deliver value for money for the state.

The meetings took place on Wednesday afternoons in Mother Superior's parlour, which was located just inside the front door of the hospital. It was a homely panelled room, which was well and expensively furnished. A trolley of freshly delivered goodies, with beautifully filled and cut sandwiches, homemade sausage rolls, coffee made with milk, china cups, the works,was available to help get us through the meeting. The Mater Hospital had been an independent hospital, funded to a great extent by football pools, until it was absorbed into the NHS in the 1960s. It had, and still has to some extent, its own particular ambience and feel. Many a morning at about eleven o'clock my mind wanders back to my Mater days when, at that time, every patient, and quite a few staff, could avail themselves of a nice bowl of homemade vegetable soup – just wonderful, and a good example of the attention to detail displayed by those who managed the hospital in those days.

Management meetings were chaired by Mother Superior, who sat at the top of the table. Also present on the particular Wednesday morning that I have in mind were Mr Casement, Mr Verzin, myself, Dr Dickie Reid – I had been a medical student with Dickie for six years and it was wonderful luck to end up working alongside him in the Mater – two midwifery sisters and the consultant anaesthetist. The pressing issues of the administration of antenatal, intrapartum (during labour) and postnatal care having been dealt with, we came to Any Other Business on the agenda. Mother Superior seemed determined, if slightly reticent, when she said that she would like to raise the issue of the 'frequent appearance of used sanitary pads littering the pavement outside the front door of the maternity unit'. She went on to say that littering of this nature had bothered her for many years, but that it was only in recent days that she felt she had the courage to mention it in public, and she wondered whether the medical staff could help to address the problem by educating our patients on etiquette in such matters, following their visits to our clinics. There was stunned silence around the table.

At this stage, it's worth detailing the local geography. If you are travelling up the Crumlin Road, the Mater Hospital is on the right-hand side, just before Crumlin Road Jail. The hospital is an imposing red-brick building with a tremendous history. For some reason, however, the maternity unit and the gynaecological unit were located across the street in terraced housing, the former unit, in particular, being in very ordinary housing indeed. In 1978 Lord Melchett, a government minister of the time, visited the maternity unit while I was working there. He was stunned when he saw the Heath Robinson contraption that we had to use in order to transfer a mother from the labour ward, down four steps and around a corner to the theatre for a Caesarean section. Within twenty-four hours of his visit, he announced that he was making six million pounds available to build a new Mater maternity unit! The great irony is that having helped to persuade Lord Melchett to make the announcement, I then spent the next thirty years trying to get government to overturn the decision to have a maternity unit on the Crumlin Road at all! As time progressed, I, along with others, became increasingly convinced that as our infrastructure improved there were huge benefits to having all our resources available in one maternity unit that was integrated into the large general hospitals. One major benefit was that transfers from Paediatrics and Intensive Care could be effected quickly and without the need for an ambulance.

The maternity unit and the gynaecology unit, therefore, were not connected – indeed there was a street and other buildings in between. Mother Superior went on to speak passionately about the women on the Shankill Road, saying, 'The strength of the women on the Shankill Road has always impressed me, as they are hard-working, courteous and grateful. I always felt I knew them well, but when I see those used sanitary towels in the street, I just wonder if my ability to assess the personality of people is wanting, as I feel that these women are letting themselves, their people, their culture and their religion down by their apparent lack of manners.' While she spoke, Joe Verzin looked shocked, Rory looked bemused, but I couldn't take my eyes off Dickie Reid, who was in convulsions of laughter. Mother Superior turned to him in mid-sentence and said, 'Doctor Reid, you may find this funny but I certainly don't. It has taken me many years to pluck up the courage to address this issue. It is a very sensitive one and I would appreciate your help rather than your attempt to turn the whole thing into a joke!' Mr Verzin chipped in and added that indeed he too had been shocked at the regularity and frequency at which these items were strewn onto the street and, although he couldn't be specific, he did notice that they seemed to litter the road more on a Thursday morning during Mr Casement's gynaecology clinic than at any other time. Well, Mr Casement wasn't too happy about that, but apart from his face taking on a bright red hue, he just kept his mouth closed. Another silence ensued, only broken by Dickie's continuous muffled laughter.

Mother Superior again said, 'We really have to do something.' To which Dickie, extracting his hankie from his mouth, said, 'Mother Superior, I have to intervene. I am not laughing at you, but you couldn't be more wrong. Could I please draw your attention to the building directly next door to the maternity unit? It is owned by Mr Nutt, the dentist. He does dental extractions on a Tuesday and Thursday morning, and then hands the patients, mostly men by the way, a Dr White's sanitary pad to jam up into their cavity to stem any residual bleeding. When his patients get outside and realise that the bleeding has stopped, they dump the towel, which just happens to be outside our door. I truly thought everyone knew that!'

There was now much relief all round. All assembled laughed and congratulated Dickie on his explanation. Mr Casement though, beamed from ear to ear, Mr Verzin gently smiled and Mother Superior probably decided to keep every other concern she ever had to herself forever.

Just a nice wee job

When I started to study medicine in 1967, only 15 per cent of my student year was female. I was aware that it was much tougher for women to succeed in the medical profession than their male counterparts, but I also had some very direct experience of one pioneering female figure within the profession in Belfast.

I was delivered in 1948 by Joy Darling (née Pedlow), a female doctor whom my mother adored. Joy was born in Belfast in 1896. She wanted to train as a doctor at Queen's University in Belfast but her father told her that 'medical school [was] no place for a woman'. She was therefore encouraged to study languages, but by translating private documents at night she was able to raise enough money to put herself through medicine. To qualify as a doctor, one had to do a significant amount of training in hospital even if the eventual aim was to be a General Practitioner. Hospitals were full of male doctors who were often compassionate, charismatic, academically brilliant, skilled, industrious and successful, but who could also be bullying, chauvinistic and self-righteous. It was a challenge for any woman to put up with such a working environment for the required four and a half years (out of a total of seven) before qualifying.

Once qualified, Joy developed a special interest in obstetrics and anaesthesia, and a particular interest in how anaesthetic agents could be used to help mothers during labour. To a great extent, she was self-taught in anaesthesia, though her expertise in the subject was eventually recognised by the Royal College of Surgeons in Ireland who presented her with an honorary degree in the subject before she retired in 1960.

At the same time that she was practising as a doctor, Joy opened a nursing home on the Antrim Road in Belfast near the city centre, providing a charitable sanctuary for young women who were pregnant but unmarried, and for injured soldiers returning from the Second World War. To help to fund the home, she offered private obstetric care for those who could afford it. As if this wasn't enough of a challenge, she also had a busy family life looking after her three children. This was how the Big Society worked at that time.

Thankfully, women nowadays do not have to struggle as much as Joy to succeed in the medical profession. Faculties of medicine throughout much of Europe, including the UK and Ireland, have a clear majority of women in their student body. Faculties with 65 to 70 per cent of women are the norm. Even more importantly, women are not just gaining places in medical school but, certainly in the UK and Ireland, are also rising swiftly through the ranks and becoming consultants and leaders within their specialities. Obstetrics and gynaecology now has 80 per cent female trainees and women account for 50 per cent of the consultants in that area. This field, in particular, used to be considered unsuitable for a woman since the hours were long, and therefore it would be impossible to be a housewife/homemaker at the same time. In addition, the fundamental aim of an obstetrician is to deliver a baby when nature falters. This was a very physically demanding job and it was considered by some that women did not possess enough physical strength for the work. However, the physical demands of the job have lessened – the emphasis on birthing mechanisms has evolved over the years and the mantra of 'a vaginal birth at almost all costs' is now rarely proclaimed by exponents of childbirth. Not only have obstetric patients changed in their expectations, requirements and choices, the same applies to gynae patients.

Men, even if not present, used to dominate gynae consultations. Back in the 70s and 80s, for example, if a woman wanted to be sterilised we had to get not only the patient to sign the consent form, but also the husband! Of course, when a man wanted a vasectomy his wife was not involved at any level!

A couple came to see me in the early 1980s at a gynae clinic to request a sterilisation procedure for the woman. In those days if you saw a male sitting in the waiting area, you just knew it was for that reason as at that time men rarely accompanied their partners to the clinic. Almost all gynae issues were seen as the preserve of the woman: infertility, menstrual disorders, sexual competency, sexually transmitted diseases and so forth – all were addressed with little, if any, male input. Nowadays, there are almost as many men as women in the waiting area.

I counselled the couple that came to see me appropriately, informing them of all the pros and cons and, with everything seemingly in order, we all signed the sterilisation consent form. My next patient was an unaccompanied woman, who also requested a sterilisation procedure. Her case was strong: seven children, age thirty-five, a smoker and accepting of the fact that while the procedure was intended to be permanent, there was a risk of surgical failure. All seemed in order. I opened the drawer and removed a consent form and completed it. The patient signed her part, and then I slipped the form into her chart and said, 'Now, when you come in your husband will have to accompany you so that he can sign the form.' She looked at me and said, 'That's not going to be possible because he's not around much and doesn't agree anyway.' I said, 'Well, those are the rules', to which she retorted indignantly, 'Well, you agreed to sterilise my friend who was in just before me.' I probably shouldn't have, but in the heat of battle I said, 'Ah yes, but her husband did sign the form.' She looked at me as if I was a few cards short of a deck and said quietly and earnestly 'And you believed her that he was her husband?'

I do remember another case in which a female patient gave

me consent to perform a procedure, albeit in a roundabout way. Mary Black was a fifty-five-year-old mother of three on whom I was to perform a vaginal hysterectomy. Mary was fit, healthy and active. However she was also naturally coy and reticent when talking about her intimate life. I had suggested that while I was performing the surgery, I could perhaps do a little bit of pelvic floor repair from which she and her husband might benefit. Mary blushed, looked sideways and scrunched up a handful of the sheets of the bed in which she was resting. I took that as a probable 'No thank you', and completed my consenting procedure. Or so I thought.

The next morning Mary was wheeled into theatre by the team while I was scrubbing up prior to the surgery. Once anaesthetised, Mary was put into the appropriate position for her surgery. At that time in that hospital there was a particular emphasis on making sure that the correct patient was having the correct surgery. Apparently in the past some patient had not had the full surgical procedure that she was expecting, resulting in a second visit to the theatre having to be scheduled. In order to try to avoid such an occurrence recurring, the theatre sister had introduced a policy whereby the patient, his or herself, wrote their name and desired operation in felt tip pen on the relevant part of their body, so that the surgeon could be in no doubt as to what he or she was to be doing, and on whom. From where I was scrubbing I could eventually see that Mary had indeed written her name on the inside of her thigh, accompanied by a description of the procedure she was supposed to have. However, I could also see that there was something written on her other thigh, but from where I stood, the words weren't visible. All did become clear when I entered the theatre and walked towards Mary. Written on her other thigh was the phrase, 'Oh to be 18 again'. Well, she may have been coy yesterday, I thought to myself, but obviously an evening lying in a gynae ward chatting to all the other patients pre- and post-operative, had obviously made her think a bit. She probably also found it easier to write her consent rather than verbalise it. I took her written observation as request and consent, and proceeded accordingly!

Male chauvinism was rife in my profession while I was doing my training but it was probably most obvious in the operating theatre. In the 1970s and the 80s, most gynaecological surgical operating lists comprised at least three or four hysterectomies. In its heyday a hysterectomy was a life-saving procedure and great skill was required to carry it out. In the resourced world, the need to perform a hysterectomy, or removal of the uterus or womb, is a skill that many gynaecologists are losing, as other surgical or medical alternatives which address equally well the gynae problems encountered have replaced this major operation.

The operation can be performed in two ways: the uterus can be removed abdominally through an incision in the woman's abdomen, or it can be removed through the vagina, with the latter operation generally being considered less invasive, and providing a shorter stay in hospital and a quicker recovery time. Indeed nowadays it is not unusual for a woman to go home less than twenty-four hours after such surgery.

It is fair to say that colleagues found that some uteri were easier to remove vaginally than others, and some gynaecologists seemed to experience a particular buzz when they removed a particularly difficult one. Those surgeons who performed vaginal hysterectomies best had legendary status, and were well aware of the fact. I assisted at one hysterectomy with a brilliant surgeon who was also known for being a bit of a male chauvinist. At this particular operation, which took place in the 1970s, there was a crowd of medical students and junior doctors in attendance.

The surgeon was performing the hysterectomy with his usual flare and aplomb, when he glanced around and caught a glimpse, out of the corner of his eye, of a young woman standing at the back of the theatre. He looked up at me briefly and said, 'What's that there?' For a second or two, I thought he was talking about a surgical landmark and I queried this with him, but he said, 'No, what's that there standing behind me over towards the door?' I looked around and saw a female medical student standing about ten feet back. I am not sure if she had heard him – I hope she hadn't.

She was wearing a completely shapeless theatre dress, a mini, in keeping with the fashion at the time. She had fairly pale legs, white bobby socks and borrowed, much-too-large, clogs on her feet. Her appearance was fairly bland and she looked scared stiff. In fairness, trainees often found themselves observing and working in theatres where they felt they almost needed permission to breathe. Invariably, someone, either the surgeon or the theatre sister, would comment at some time throughout the session that they were inappropriately dressed or standing in the wrong place. I whispered in the consultant's ear, 'She is a young medical student, sir'. He carried on operating with great speed and skill, and commented, 'We better train that well.' I suspected what he meant but I couldn't believe he had said it. I whispered, 'Why is that, sir?' His response was immediate and said it all, 'It looks like it will be in medicine for a long time.' In one statement he had decided that she was an 'it', unattractive, unlikely to get married, and as a result, unlikely to bear children, and would therefore be in medicine for the long term.

Things did change but it was a slow process. My memory is that it was around 1970 before the first female consultant in the main corridor of our hospital was appointed, a fact that is even more extraordinary when you consider that we were in the largest teaching hospital in Northern Ireland. The majority of women who qualified in medicine in the 1970s and 1980s went into family planning, ultrasound, dermatology or laboratory medicine, and the posts were quite openly referred to as, 'a nice wee job for a woman'. It is to my own shame that at that time, some forty years ago, I saw nothing wrong with that description, and it was my impression that the women who were lucky enough to obtain these 'nice wee jobs' were happy with their lot.

The women who took such posts as I have described were vocationally driven. It would take a future generation of women, equally vocationally driven, but supported by society in general, to rattle the heavily armoured but far from gilded cage of medicine.

Mum says you saved my life

I went to the antenatal clinic in Jubilee Maternity Hospital, Belfast, one Monday morning in 1982. I was then a senior registrar and therefore worked along with the consultant, who was at this time, Ken Houston. This responsibility and honour meant that I saw mothers who had been identified as being high risk or were booking in officially to our maternity unit for the first time in their current pregnancy. Mary Grant, who I was scheduled to see, fell into the latter category.

By the time the consultant or I saw a new booker at the antenatal clinic, they had already provided a lot of information to the booking midwife, and the clerical staff would have prepared a chart. In the 1970s and 80s you could tell a great deal about a patient by looking just at the front of the chart – her age, probable ethnicity, where she lived, her husband's occupation (which also tended to be a marker of social class back then), the number of pregnancies (both successful and unsuccessful) she had experienced, her blood group, and the date of her last menstrual period. A quick glance inside the first page of the chart gave me a summary of the past medical and family history, as well as any other key factors appropriate to the current pregnancy, including levels of smoking, alcohol consumption and fitness. By the time I met the woman in question I certainly believed I knew quite a lot about her and her background.

Mary's chart told me that she was booking in for her first pregnancy and that she was about eighteen weeks pregnant.

The only unusual feature to strike me was that she lived in Banbridge, which is about twenty miles away from Belfast. That was quite far away for a mother booking into the Jubilee, which was situated almost in the centre of Belfast. At that time there were over thirty places in Northern Ireland in which to give birth outside the home (there are now nine and probably should be five). I wondered what it was that had encouraged Mary to disregard the two maternity units that were nearer her to come to the Jubilee.

Having introduced myself, I asked her that very question. Her answer was that it was 'because of Mr Houston'. She went on, 'I was my mother's first baby and she tells me that Mr Houston delivered me one winter's night in 1960. Mum said she had been in labour a very long time when Mr Houston arrived like a knight on a white horse and saved her life, and gave her the wee treasure she always wanted. That's me by the way. Not so wee now!' We had a good laugh together and I promised that I would introduce her to Mr Houston before she left the clinic. She blushed at the thought. I carried out an examination and found her to have a very healthy pregnancy. I then told her to sit in the waiting room while I went to find Mr Houston.

Ken was sitting at a desk in the coffee room having his staple diet – in those days at least – of coffee and Gallagher's Blues cigarettes. I said to him, 'Tell me this, twenty-two years ago, when you were working in the Lagan Valley Hospital in Lisburn, do you remember delivering Beryl Richmond, and saving her baby?' He told me he hadn't been working at Lagan Valley twenty-two years ago. I told him, "There's a woman in the waiting room who says that you delivered her in 1960, and she has come back to have her baby delivered by you because her mum tells her you saved her life. She's 100 per cent sure it was you.' His eyes then lit up as he suddenly remembered and said, 'Jim. She is correct, I remember now. Was it in the winter?' I told him it was – Mary was born on 14 January 1960.

There clearly was a real story to be told about Mary's birth, and Ken started to tell me it. 'I remember it completely, but before I go on, how is she?' I said she was great, that she had attended grammar school and then worked in the bank until she got married. She was now expecting her first child and all seemed to be going well in the pregnancy. 'Why do you ask?' I said. Ken smiled. 'Wait till you hear about that birth, and then you'll understand. It all started on a Saturday afternoon. I was working here in Jubilee and was the senior registrar on call. In those days there weren't many of us about – there only were about ten consultants in the whole of Northern Ireland, and about five of us were all hanging about waiting for dead men's shoes. In the 1950s and '60s, the senior registrar here covered the Samaritan Hospital, the Gardner Robb, the Jubilee Hospital, Malone Place and Lagan Valley – that's five delivery suites.

'The first four of those units were all very close together, within a mile of each other, but Lagan Valley was a good ten miles away. In those days, not too long after the National Health Service first started, it was a lot easier to open a maternity hospital than to close one. Communications and the road networks were poor and women had scarce enough access to transport. Maternity units at that time didn't need much in the way of high-tech equipment, and so any moderately sized building could easily be converted and renamed a "nursing home". They were very busy units too, and were an oasis for many mothers who, quite honestly, often lived in very average surroundings and found themselves pregnant with alarming frequency.

'GPs did a lot of deliveries at Lagan Valley and at Malone Place, but if they got into trouble they had to ring us. I was on duty with the famous Mr Joe Watt, but needless to say he was at home on the Malone Road.' At that time, there weren't too many gynaecologists around, but the ones that were worked very hard for the NHS, had flourishing private practices, but covered huge geographical areas when they were on call. Of course prior to the inception of the NHS they also worked extremely hard, and much of their work was performed as an act of charity. Sometimes the consultant would be needed in

Ballymena, which was thirty-five miles away from Belfast, and not serviced by particularly good roads. They could be halfway there, at a landmark such as Corr's Corner, when the police would stop the car at a road block and inform the consultant that the patient they were going to see had died, and then ask him to head to Dungannon, fifty miles away in the other direction, as 'they have a woman there who needs your help doctor'.

Mr Watt was a legendary figure within gynaecological circles. No matter how busy he was, he was always immaculately dressed, day or night. They say that he could be called at three o'clock in the morning and he would come into the labour ward perfectly turned out. Some believed that he had a magic razor that just glided across his face every half hour throughout the night, and he always had a starched collar, a perfectly knotted tie, and his hair immaculately Brylcreemed to the right.

That Sunday in January, Mr Watt was at home. Ken had been dealing with a severe case of maternal haemorrhage following childbirth and had eventually managed to get things under control. 'The sister then came and asked me to look at a patient who had a case of deep transverse arrest. It was pretty obvious that I was going to have to take the patient to theatre to attempt a forceps delivery, but before I could even get there, there was a call from Gardner Robb to say that they had a case that was very similar. Just when I put the phone down, it rang again to say that there was a similar case of deep transverse arrest in the Samaritan Hospital at the other side of the Lisburn Road. I decided to gird my loins and have another cup of tea with three spoonfuls of sugar in it this time [a euphemism for a cigarette!] Halfway through that – I could hardly believe it – but the sister at Lagan Valley Hospital rang to say that there was woman who had been pushing for two hours and there was still no sign of the baby. I told her I would be back in touch when I could. I knew that none of these maternity units had staff capable of carrying out the procedures that would be required. I decided that if I did the one in Jubilee first, even if I had to do a Caesarean, once the baby was out, the senior house officer could take over and finish the procedure.

'It wasn't often that we called in the consultant – senior registrars in those days were meant to be consultants-in-waiting, and indeed we were. There were big interviews looming and you definitely did not want to give the impression, which could be widely disseminated, that you weren't up to the mark and couldn't cope under pressure. So, it was with slight trepidation that I phoned Joe Watt on a Sunday afternoon in the middle of winter in 1960. He came to the phone and I said, "Ken Houston here, Mr Watt". We exchanged pleasantries and then I said to him "Mr Watt, I was wondering if you could give me some help". He answered positively and said, "Anything I can do, I will, I would be more than happy to give you help, Ken." I said, "It's like this, Mr Watt, I am talking to you from Jubilee labour ward, and I have a case of a primigravida with a deep transverse arrest. She has been pushing two hours now and she's a spent force. I think I should take her to theatre." Mr Watt intervened and said, "Absolutely, Ken, it's the right thing to do, no doubt. I know you are well capable of that. You get on with it." I then interjected, "The only problem is I think I may need your help as I was about to go and do that case when I received phone calls from Gardner Robb, the Samaritan and Lagan Valley to say that they have mothers with the same problem." There was a five-second silence on the phone, then he said, "You need my help, don't you, Ken?" I said, "I would really appreciate that greatly." After another pause of maybe a full three seconds he said, "Well, since you are in Jubilee, I think you should do that one first, then I think you should go over to the Samaritan and you would probably be best to take someone who can give the anaesthetic with you. When you have got that one sorted, I would head over to Gardner Robb and by the time you make it out to Lagan Valley [ten miles away in the snow, A-class roads only], you will probably find that the woman has delivered, so I suggest you phone them before you go, just to see how the land lies. I hope that advice is helpful."

'I was stunned, but after about five seconds silence from me this time, I came up with, "Thank you very much, Mr Watt, that is indeed very helpful, I will let you know if things don't work out as you have suggested." I put the phone down and thought a very bad word indeed.

'I took the woman in the Jubilee to theatre and incredibly the baby just wouldn't come the traditional route, so we did a Caesarean section. The whole thing took a couple of hours. I then went across to Gardner Robb and the woman there still wasn't delivered so I attempted a forceps delivery. Again the baby wouldn't come, so we did another Caesarean. That took another two hours. We then went over to the Samaritan and, believe it or not, did the same thing again.

'At the end of all that I rang Lagan Valley and I said, "Sister, please tell me that your patient has delivered." She said, "I'm afraid not, Mr Houston. She is beyond herself." I told her I would be with them soon. I got into my Morris Minor and trundled up the Lisburn Road. The snow was getting heavier and I was pretty exhausted, but at least getting into the car gave me a chance to have a couple of fags.

'By the time I arrived, I could see that everybody was exhausted. I remember thinking that I couldn't do another Caesarean section – in those days the consultants killed you for doing a Caesarean section that wasn't needed. It was a big blot on your copybook. I was thinking through each of the three attempts that I had made to achieve a traditional route birth. I had never had a situation like that before in my life and I decided that I couldn't live with having to do four Caesarean sections in a row. So by the time I went to see Beryl Richmond, I had decided in my, mind that, come what may, that baby was coming out the direction it had started pointing. I don't really remember a lot about Mrs Richmond personally, but I remember that once I got the forceps on, I decided this baby was coming out pointing south. It was a difficult enough delivery, not too bad though, but out she came and she cried immediately. And that, Jim, is the woman who is sitting out there.'

Ken was a great storyteller and probably the most caring, empathetic man with whom I ever worked. First and foremost, he loved women. As he got up and stubbed out his cigarette, he passed some comment about Joe Watt that I really didn't hear, but it would have been unlikely to be a direct quote from his eulogy.

Mary blushed to the roots of her hair again when she met Ken and he beamed from cheek to cheek. She gave him a big hug and said, 'Oh thank you, Mr Houston. Mum said you saved my life, and hers.' In the context of 1960, she was just about right.

The flying squad

Until very recently, all major hospitals in the UK had access to an obstetric flying squad. The flying squad was a special ambulance that was called out in cases of maternity problems. When everything is going smoothly, childbirth seems like one of the most natural things in the world. But when a birth goes wrong, things can become very serious very fast. And things can go wrong very, very quickly. With that in mind, the whole country had access to these flying squads,which comprised an ambulance with experienced ambulance drivers, a midwife, a trainee obstetrician, and a suitcase full of instruments, drugs and equipment.

The flying squad responded rapidly to calls from GPs, or indeed members of the public, who rang the maternity unit in question directly. Bleeding (haemorrhage) from the birth canal before, after or during birth was number one on the list of reported problems. When the call came in, the crew and ambulance would go out at breakneck speed and deal with the problem at the patient's house, stabilise her, and then bring her back to the hospital. With improved communications, roads, and antenatal care, far fewer unexpected disasters occur nowadays, and when they do, these improvements mean that the best course of action for any woman is usually to get herself to her local maternity unit as quickly as possible by her own methods. In 1976 things weren't like that.

Roisin Maguire lived in Whitehead, a beautiful seaside

town on the edge of Belfast Lough, about forty minutes drive from Belfast. Her GP phoned us in the labour ward at 6 a.m. one morning, ten days after she had given birth via a forceps delivery to a healthy baby girl at the Jubilee Maternity Hospital. Roisin had suffered a fairly large and totally unexpected bleed from her birth canal, and while her family doctor had managed to administer the appropriate drugs to stabilise her condition, Roisin obviously needed to come back into hospital so that we could address the underlying problem.

I was the obstetrician on duty with the flying squad that morning and, along with the midwife Daphne, I shot down to the front door of the unit to be met by the ambulance and drivers, Fred and John. Fred asked, 'Is this the real thing, or a fag and bag call, doctor?' I told him that I thought it was the real thing, but I understood what he meant. Often the flying squad was called out and when they arrived at the address in question, the woman who had requested the service would be standing at the front door of her house, with her handbag over one arm and a cigarette on the go. These women had certainly learnt how to work the system. In those days transport wasn't easily obtained in the middle of the night – most families didn't own a car and taxis were for very rich people. The best way to get to hospital was to ring for the flying squad.

We made our way to Whitehead at a good rate of knots. Having raced out of Belfast City Hospital and grounds and past Belfast City Hall and joined the main road out of the city, there then was a calmer atmosphere, and John turned to me and said, 'Doc, have a look around you, and you will see that this ambulance isn't like any other.' I noticed that some things did indeed look a bit unusual. Way ahead of its time, there was resuscitative equipment including breathing masks, Ambu bags (for pumping air into the lungs), a portable defibrillator to get hearts back into normal rhythm (which had been invented in Belfast by Professor Frank Pantridge) and an array of bandages, splints and tubing all tied up in clear plastic bags around the interior. John went on, 'You see, Doc, this is Fred and mine's ambulance, and we are the only ones that drive it. We have just been just been away on a six-week course on anatomy, physiology and all diseases, and we are now ready to cope with everything.' I told John that I was very impressed by the instruments and labelling on display in the ambulance – it really did look like the medical equivalent of a one-man band. I was also impressed by John's eloquence and by his perhaps slightly ambitious belief that they could now 'cope with everything' following his six-week course. The mid- to late-1970s, however, marked the beginning of paramedics really becoming involved in medicine and increasingly proving that they were capable of doing much more than just providing a method of fast transport between incident and hospital. John and Fred were part of that. Our paramedical colleagues are capable of just as much as many doctors and nurses, and indeed more than most doctors and nurses when it comes to their specialised areas.

After about twenty-five minutes of pretty fast driving we arrived at Roisin's address in Whitehead. I knew Roisin from her time in the Jubilee for the birth of her baby – in those days patients used to stay in for quite a few days and you got to know them. Nowadays, the vast majority of women are discharged within six hours of giving birth, so medical staff don't have the opportunity to build a relationship with them. When we got to the bedside, Daphne checked Roisin's observations and found her to be stable. I gave her a quick examination and it was clear that we weren't in an acute situation. The GP's actions had been totally appropriate and the situation was stable. Roisin was obviously quite frightened by the appearance of so much blood just at the time when she was getting over a forceps delivery. Her concern and fears were well justified – it is said that three jumbo jets full of women die every day in Africa alone from bleeding after childbirth.

Mostly, this bleeding is caused by the womb not contracting down hard after the placenta is expelled. This happens in an unfairly large proportion of cases. Incredibly, if any trained birth attendant is standing by they can often stop the bleeding simply by massaging the womb. The second reason the womb bleeds after delivery is because the human placenta is made up of twenty or so mini placentas (cotyledons) and one or two can be left behind after expulsion and it is nobody's fault. Nature is amazing, but the process of ridding the mother of the placenta after birth is obviously a work in progress. It's the one part of childbirth in the human that should be very straightforward but, sadly, 'leaving it to nature alone' can have catastrophic consequences on too many occasions.

I have always been sympathetic to the effect this apparent clinical catastrophe of bleeding after childbirth has on mothers. As adults we all know to use pressure or a tourniquet to control bleeding, but when there is no logical or obvious way to stop the blood literally pouring from you, and at the same time you feel your very life ebbing away, the terrible helplessness and loss of confidence mothers experience stay with them for a very long time afterwards.

Roisin was, however, reassured by the sight of us all in the room, particularly when we told her that we thought the problem was simply that a piece of the placenta was probably still in her uterus and that we only needed to bring her back to the hospital for twelve to twenty-four hours. (I remember a woman coming in with the same problem, which we dealt with. Before discharging her, I explained that we had removed a piece of placenta that had been left in her uterus after childbirth. She interrupted me. 'No problem, doctor, I know myself how busy they were that night in the labour ward. It's perfectly understandable that a thing like that should happen!' Sometimes we have to take the flack for nature's slip-ups!)

Fred and John strapped Roisin into an ambulance chair and carried her into the back of the vehicle, and then made her comfortable on the stretcher. The baby stayed at home with Roisin's husband, as was more the norm in those days. We reassured him that all was going to be well, and having thanked the GP for a timely call, Daphne and I climbed into the back of the ambulance to be with Roisin.

As we drove out onto the main road, I was quite taken aback by the speed we were doing. We had the siren on and the light flashing, and Fred seemed to be doing a fairly good impression of Paddy Hopkirk, the local world champion rally driver, as he went round the country roads. Daphne was continuing to take observations and I was chatting to Roisin. She seemed extremely stable and looked very well. But it became apparent to me that Fred and John knew something we didn't, as we just kept going faster and faster.

As we hit the main road Fred's foot really went to the board. I looked at Daphne, looked at the patient, and looked back at Daphne, and we both wondered if we were missing something and if there really was a need to go at this speed. As we drove into the centre of Belfast, the ambulance went about as fast as was safely possible. A quick glance at the patient showed no obvious deterioration. The ambulance then, rather than going back to the Jubilee, continued to travel in the direction of the Royal Victoria Hospital. I commented on this to Fred and he said, 'Yes, that's right, doctor.' I said nothing more. Fred was in complete charge. I was obviously only along for the ride, albeit a white-knuckle one. We sped through the roundabouts towards the Royal, but then the maternity unit became a vision in the rearview mirror as we sped past it! What was going on?

Suddenly we screeched to an unexpected halt outside the Belfast ambulance depot. Fred turned around to me and said, 'Okay, Doc, that's it, our shift is over, there will be another crew out in a few minutes to take you over to the Jubilee.' Daphne, Roisin and I looked at each other and could only smile. I looked at my watch – it was one minute to eight in the morning. Right enough, his shift was over.

The next fresh-faced shift of two well rested crewmen came out and we drove over to the Jubilee at a steady pace. Roisin was taken to the labour ward and treated and was back in Whitehead the next day.

The recent 'progress' towards all healthcare providers working in tightly regulated shifts has been a bit of a shock to us of the older generation. Fred and John were just ahead of their time by about thirty years. A retired consultant recently asked me if young people were going into medicine today as a vocation or as a job. The question is not easily answered and I can't and shouldn't generalise, but certainly I have noticed a major shift in attitude among healthcare providers in recent years. There was a great feeling in the past that the NHS was *ours*, our baby, where we could practise our skills, be reasonably rewarded, do good, have a bit of craic and come home when we had finished our work. Now, the NHS feels as though it's *theirs*, and we are employed in shifts to work it for *them*. Again, I am generalising but morale is frequently low, and that didn't happen by chance. The place of the NHS has – to some extent, and especially for those of us of a passing generation – moved from holding a place in our heart to holding a place in our head. The answer to the question, 'Who should be in control in the NHS in the future?' seems to have been discussed and decided some time ago, and at a much higher place than the labour ward floor or the back of an ambulance.

A wee form

It was 1976. I had qualified as a doctor in 1973 and, as part of my houseman's year, I was working in Jubilee 4, the neonatal unit of Belfast City Hospital, under a wonderful pioneering woman, Dr Muriel Frazer. She was a paediatrician who was deeply sceptical about the intentions of most of the obstetricians she met. In fact, she often said that obstetricians treated babies as toxic by-products of pregnancy! I didn't and don't agree with her view. It appeared to me that in the 1960s and '70s obstetricians were only just getting to the stage at which, in the developed world, women had a fair chance of making it out of a pregnancy alive. Quite naturally, the major focus of maternity care at that time was the mother.

Working with Dr Frazer, however, did give me an opportunity to be at many normal, and quite a few not-so-normal, deliveries and I was quickly smitten by my work in the maternity unit. When you hear a newborn baby cry and realise that it nearly might not have done so, it is an overwhelming feeling and its effects stay with you forever. In those days, practical learning was gained mostly by experience. There was not so much preventive medicine around and many pregnancies were complicated by maternal rheumatic heart disease, anaemia, and chest complaints, never mind that most of the emergencies we dealt with in the labour ward were totally unexpected. There was a lot to be learned by us young trainees in maternity units, and the time we put in was extensive, to say the least.

Working between 100 and 128 hours a week was pretty common. Learning on the job is going out of fashion now as, thanks to the EWTD (European Working Time Directive), it's illegal to work more than 45 hours per week. Much learning is acquired by simulation exercises and computer models, and there is of course much to be said for this type of learning. The airline industry is often presented to us as an example of how we should proceed, and our attention is drawn to how pilots can be trained to land their plane on water without actually having to do so. Mind you, the comparison doesn't hold so well when we are rushed off our feet in the labour ward. We can't just take a leaf out of the airline industry's book and say, 'sorry, due to bad weather our airport is now closed'!

I am certainly not saying that everything was great in the good old days – it wasn't. The modern skills and drills, and competency-based learning, are probably best for all concerned, but it could be even better if doctors had the opportunity to gain more experience before they were left to practise on their own. Almost all my immediate predecessors spent time working with luminaries in African and Asian countries and this allowed them to get unparalleled experience from working with hugely talented men and, occasionally, women who were carrying out fantastic work in the emerging nations of that continent. In return, those continents got to draw on the expertise of the obstetricians and gynaecologists from our Royal Colleges. Many international trainees also got the opportunity to come to the UK for postgraduate training, and some still do. It was, and is, a win-win situation for all concerned. Unfortunately, for a range of reasons, the whole concept of UK students getting practical training in the under-resourced world disappeared in the 1980s, but many of us feel that formal trainee exchanges should be introduced. Our trainees would definitely benefit from working in truly busy clinical settings alongside extremely experienced colleagues, and international trainees would benefit from being exposed to the communication and risk-aversion agendas that have so appropriately pervaded the NHS in recent times. The bureaucratic and practical hurdles seem to be insurmountable at the moment, but as a solution for both sides, it makes perfect sense. Like so much else, it just needs the political will.

Not only have our work patterns changed over the decades, so too have the requirements of our patients. The way in which we practise obstetrics reflects the social and cultural changes that are occurring in society. Improved economies mean increasing independence for individuals and increased access to material goods – including contraception – which in turn can mean easier living. Our reproductive behaviour is a reflection of society and vice versa. The whole concept of unmarried mothers coming into hospital with their heads held high, which is now quite rightly the norm, was still some way off in 1976. Newspapers throughout Ireland at that time were peppered with stories of newborn babies being left in churchyards, on the steps of police stations, or at the local parochial house. The introduction of the 1967 Abortion Act in England and Wales had mostly, though not completely, stopped the horribly endless list of young women dying from botched abortions, but there was still quite a stigma to having a baby outside wedlock in the 1970s. The world of maternity care, and indeed the administrative system associated with it, was geared towards married couples.

It was against this background that young Emma came into our unit one Saturday night. She was unmarried and had a boyfriend, Robert. She was sassy, assured, bright and focussed. I warmed to her immediately. Her own father had died young and she had been raised by her mum, who was very supportive of the pregnancy. The tragedy was that, when Emma presented herself in labour at her due date, the baby's heartbeat could not be detected. We were all distraught: Emma, Robert, her mum, the midwives and me. Stillbirth, for no apparent cause, just seemed so unfair, and still does to this day. How could this baby who had been kicking away for forty weeks just stop?

Emma was so controlled and seemed to be there for everyone around her, rather than vice versa. She proceeded to give birth to a beautiful baby girl with no apparent external problems, though in retrospect, the baby was under-nourished and too small for that stage of pregnancy. Emma agreed that her newborn baby, Rosie, should have a postmortem the next morning. However, at about midday, I got a phone call asking that I go and see Emma. She explained to me that the mortuary had been on the phone demanding a consent form to be signed by the 'husband'. Robert had run over to the mortuary to provide the required signature, but when he got there, he was told that it had to be the mother's husband that signed the form, rather than the child's father. He was quite rightly affronted, but could make no headway with the authorities he encountered there. He returned rather sheepishly to Emma, and she asked for me to be called. Robert was a solid, good guy, and he accepted the situation, even though it was illogical as he was plainly the father of the baby. When I arrived, Emma said to me, 'Dr Dornan, could you make up a wee consent form for Robert to sign? This death means as much to him as it does to me. I want him to feel as involved officially as I am.' Such maturity, wisdom and compassion from a young woman who had just experienced a terrible trauma.

I drew up the required form and talked to the guys in the mortuary. They were a sensible bunch and quickly accepted the form that Robert would sign. The postmortem was performed and proved inconclusive, as is so often and tragically the case with stillbirths.

While attitudes towards unmarried mothers have moved on tremendously in much of the developed world, in many parts of the world a woman can still be flogged, tortured or killed for even having sex outside marriage never mind carrying a baby. But I know of *no* country that treats men the same way for the same apparent indiscretions. Not that I would want them to do so, but the inequality is just so blatant.

In my working career I have been privileged to meet many courageous and wonderful women but Emma was one of the first, a real trailblazer.

Millennium Development Goals

The Millennium Development Goals (MDGs) were announced in the year 2000, after 189 countries got together and declared set targets for global action against poverty, to be reached by the year 2015. Millennium Goals 4 and 5, which are to reduce child mortality and to improve maternal health, have particular relevance for obstetricians.

I became personally involved in international women's health in 2004 when I became Senior Vice President of the Royal College of Obstetricians and Gynaecologists in London. When I took over the post I had two responsibilities: postgraduate education and international women's health. The latter fascinated me particularly, probably because my wife is part-Afghan and we have travelled to Asia and Africa together on many occasions, and witnessed for ourselves that women in general are not in a good place in those countries. My wife is also a fine obstetrician and gynaecologist, and a supporter of the desperately necessary improvement of women's rights throughout the world.

As Senior Vice President I quickly became convinced that while it was important and worthwhile to address MDGs 4 and 5, the actual answer to these problems was MDG 3: 'To promote gender equality and the empowerment of women'. Give women the tools provided under MDG 3, and MDGs 4 and 5 will follow. The MDGs, impressive as they may be, pay little attention to dignity, human rights, violence towards women, and sexual and reproductive rights.

In 2010 I had occasion to sit beside Anne, a woman of Swedish origin, at a New Year's Eve dinner party in the west of Ireland. At the time I had just turned sixty. Anne was in her late fifties. We were reflecting on our youth and on the traits associated with our different nationalities. I told Anne that I believed that the archetypal Swedish woman was beautiful, slim, had long blonde hair, enjoyed saunas and – most importantly – had been given the freedom to make love and was generally a firm believer in gender equality. Anne agreed that much of what I had said was true, but that, far more significant than having been given the freedom to make love in the 1960s, was that she and her generation had been given the freedom *not* to make love as well. This was quite a startling statement to me, and so she went on to explain.

Her sister Helga had been a few years older than her, and while she was brought up with many freedoms, it had still been expected of her that, following tertiary education, she would marry and have children. Anne and her generation, however, who grew up a little later in the 1960s, had a strong sense that they were equal citizens with men and could choose whether to have sex or not, whether to have children or not. There was absolutely no pressure to conform to the previous model of marriage and family. I was honestly stunned by this definition of true freedom. I could see that no matter what contraception and health services were available to women worldwide, the vast, vast, vast majority did not possess or even come close to possessing that ultimate freedom of mind that Anne had described, that freedom not to have to conform to a previous generation's expectations.

Anne's situation while she was growing up was certainly quite different from that of many other women across the developed and developing world. Most women in the world are seen by men as chattels, vessels, or baby machines. The final product, the baby – preferably male – is a sign of masculinity for the man and represents the continuation of the family name and the male line. In this way, patriarchy and patrilinearity are guaranteed.

In prehistoric times matriarchy and matrilinearity were the key driving forces in society, but with the development of writing and the keeping of records, inheritance became the key issue. Men were the scribes and keepers of records and it was they who developed the various religions that ultimately and sadly demoted woman from their position as goddess with the ultimate power to give birth, to a position where the latter was being performed as a function of her being, rather than the miracle it is considered to be in pagan religions.

The male leaders of the emerging churches of the time quickly decided that patriarchy and patrilinearity should be the deciding factors when it came to inheritance and so to this day, in much of the world, the man is seen as the head of the household, and often land and property is only passed on to sons (it also explains why some churches introduced celibacy, so that there was no opportunity of church property having to be divided up on the death of the church employee).

I was absolutely fascinated by Anne's conclusion that it was just as important to have the freedom not to make love as to make love and I asked her, perhaps naively, why Sweden was so much further ahead in the 1960s and 1970s than any other European country. She looked at me with incredulity and said, 'The answer is very simple: we didn't fight wars. Countries that fight wars elevate men above others, namely women – they are either constantly preparing for men going to war, producing men to go to war, producing weapons for men to take to war, preparing for men coming back from war and either honouring their dead or, indeed, their living men.' It was all so obvious and logical. If you take testosterone and hence war out of the equation, then men and women would have a much better chance of not only being *seen* as equal in our society, but of being equal.

At the beginning of the recent millennium, many descendants

of ancient civilisations were asked how they thought modern man had coped with the past few millennia. The Native American Indians were asked what their reflections were on the world in the three or four thousand years since history started being written down. In their conclusion they used the American native language word 'Koyaanisqatsi', which means 'life out of balance'. Their very strong feeling was that, on reflection, the last three thousand years had been similar to an experiment in patriarchy, and that it had been filled with testosterone-fuelled wars, and that it had been a time when men's egos had been running wildly and untethered. For them, the last three millennia had seen the creation of a plethora of misogynistic societies and human beings had shown a huge disrespect for mother earth. These reflections convinced me even more that MDG 3, the promotion of gender equality and empowerment of women through education, needs to be addressed before the proposed deadline in 2015. But I don't think this will happen. The will would need to be there, and it is not. Yet.

One in two hundred

One statistic that is universally accepted is that in one in two hundred pregnancies, the implantation of the fertilised egg occurs too low down in the uterus, meaning that the placenta ends up lying in front of the baby, partly or completely blocking the birth canal. This is known as placenta (afterbirth) praevia (in front) and, if the mother is left to go into labour in a non-clinical environment, without any skilled birth attendant in the vicinity, both she and the baby will die. This is 'nature at its worst'. There is simply no action that human beings can take anywhere on this planet to prevent placenta praevia occurring in at least one in two hundred pregnancies. It just happens, and the outcome in non-clinical environments is catastrophic. It is sobering to remember that *over half* the women in the world still deliver in non-clinical surroundings.

For those who give birth in a clinical environment, methods of addressing placenta praevia have evolved over time. In the days before Caesarean sections became a very acceptable and safe alternative to vaginal delivery, obstetricians developed manoeuvres and procedures for trying to save the mother's life at all cost. For the vast majority of obstetricians in the world, the mother's life is sacred and, indeed, *salus matris suprema lex* or 'the mother's life is sacred' is embedded in UK law. In many Western countries, such as Canada, some Catholic maternity institutions were perceived to have the view that the baby's life was even more sacred or at least equal to that of the mother, and indeed many mothers attended these institutions out of choice, as they valued the life of their newborn above their own. Some women still choose to deliver in a setting where they know that – if a choice is to be made by the carer as to whose life to save in a 50:50 situation – the carer will save the baby, at the potential expense of the mother's life.

In previous generations in the developed world, many women went through pregnancy in the knowledge that it could well be a death sentence rather than a time of great joy. This experience may be a thing of the past in the West, but it is still the situation for many women in the under-resourced world. For example, the maternal mortality rates in rural Afghanistan, and it is by no means unique, reveal that a woman who has six children has a staggering lifetime risk of one in six of dying during pregnancy.

When I came into obstetrics in the 1970s, avoiding doing a Caesarean section at almost all costs within institutions in the Western world was very much the order of the day. Obstetricians often used the word 'failure' when describing an indication for performing a Caesarean section, as in failed forceps, failed vacuum, failed breech, failed trial of scar, failed trial of labour. All were terms whose inference was 'failed obstetrician'. He (invariably he) had failed to find a way of delivering the baby through the birth canal.

I have already mentioned the debate that rages around the issue of Caesareans. However, that aside, everyone now agrees that there are occasions when a Caesarean section is the best route for mother and baby, and placenta praevia is one of them. But it wasn't always like that. A non-surgical technique for managing a woman with placenta praevia was popular with obstetricians and midwives in the early part of the twentieth century and before, but it normally involved sacrificing the fetal life in order to preserve the maternal life. As term approaches, and the uterus (womb) prepares itself for the birthing process, the lower part begins to thin and to be drawn up into the upper pelvis with the aim of letting the baby move downwards. If the placenta is attached in part or completely to this lower segment, it shears away from the lower segment and serious bleeding can occur. This bleeding may be torrential and mothers, and hence their babies also, can die in minutes from blood loss.

Attendants who were either trying to avoid Caesarean section or were not in a situation where the life-saving operation could be performed, introduced their fingers and hand into the birth canal, and through the cervix. They would then push through the placenta itself and get hold of the baby's foot, while helping to externally spin the baby round with their other hand. The aim was then to pull one of the baby's legs through the cervix, exteriorising it. Weights were subsequently secured to the foot and tied to a line over the end of the bed, so that the pressure of the baby's buttocks on the lower segment of the womb hugely reduced the loss of maternal blood and thus prevented the mother dying from haemorrhage. In the fullness of time labour would ensue, and bring with it the birth of the baby, who was very probably but not always dead, but the mother's life would usually be preserved. The scenario sounds brutal, and it was to an extent, but at least it saved the mother's life rather than both lives being lost.

My hometown of Belfast is famous obstetrically for producing a man who turned the approach to antenatal haemorrhage on its head. His name was Charles Horner Greer Macafee and he was Head of the Department of Midwifery and Gynaecology at Queen's University from 1945 to 1963. He was one of the first people to put forward the idea that when a mother bleeds before birth, it should not necessarily be seen as a dire emergency requiring immediate intervention. Instead he suggested that a conservative approach could be considered: the bleeding would often settle by itself, at least for a short time, enough time to allow the baby to mature. The key platforms of Macafee's theory required that the mother should be kept in the hospital at all times and that any anaemia should be corrected by the use of blood products or iron. Within the maternity unit in which the mother was a patient, there should permanently be personnel on hand with the ability to perform a Caesarean section at very short notice and the plan should be to get the baby almost to term.

Meanwhile, efforts should be made to determine where the placenta was so that a decision regarding delivery could be made. Sometimes all is not what it seems! Clinically, the history and physical findings may suggest placenta praevia, but imaging techniques sometimes tell otherwise. In the past we used to talk of the 'migrating placenta', suggesting that the placenta moves in pregnancy. However, it doesn't physically move. It simply appears to move, for as the lower part of the womb stretches upwards in the last months of pregnancy to allow the fetal head to descend, the placenta rises up with it. The agreed final precise site of the placenta can be in some doubt until the last minute. If the placenta is still low when the time comes to give birth, a Caesarean section should be carried out, but if the placenta has 'moved up' with the developing lower segment, then a vaginal birth is possible.

Macafee's conservative approach to the management of placenta praevia remains the standard one in institutionalised obstetrics across the world. As with many great men, the timing of Macafee's astute observations and resultant treatise was as important as the idea itself. Macafee's approach came serendipitously at the same time that the increasing safety of the Caesarean section procedure was being observed, and when specialist anaesthetists and paediatricians with an interest in the newborn were becoming increasingly involved in pregnancy and birth.

While medicine continues to move forward at a great pace, it is often worthwhile to remind the next generation of the trials and tribulations endured by previous generations. Teaching at the bedside used to be a great way of doing this, as well as being beneficial in so many other ways, but sadly it has just about disappeared from medical training in the UK and Ireland.

In the late 1970s I was a registrar and was carrying out a teaching ward round with half a dozen medical students in a local hospital. Among the medical students was a young woman, Rhonda, who was one of these dynamic young people who made a lasting impact on those around them. I noticed her straight away. Not only was she a female student, unusual enough in the late 1970s, but she also didn't lack confidence or attitude.

We stopped at the bedside of a patient who was thirty-six weeks pregnant, was confirmed to have placenta praevia, had bled heavily on three occasions during her eight-week stay in hospital, and was just waiting another couple of weeks for her Caesarean section. I informed the students of all the important elements of this conservative management technique, but I also informed them of the heroics and manipulations performed in 'historic times'. Rhonda interrupted me and said, 'I know exactly what you are talking about. My sister was delivered by Professor Macafee in the way you have just described.' I was stunned because I thought the method of delivery was long since redundant. Rhonda told us what had happened: 'Mummy was a patient of Professor Macafee's before he came up with his idea of conservative management. When she was about eight months pregnant, she came into the hospital as an emergency because she was bleeding. Professor Macafee examined my mother just as you described and determined that the placenta was indeed low. My mother was apparently doing her best to bleed to death. Professor Macafee, just as you described, inserted his hand through Mummy's birth canal under anaesthetic, through her cervix and through the placenta, and grabbed hold of my sister's foot. He tied a weight to my sister's leg, just as you described, and sure enough my mother did stop bleeding. Professor Macafee then woke Mummy up from the anaesthetic and told her that she would now have to labour, that hopefully she wouldn't bleed any more, but that her baby would probably die in the process. After about six hours the baby was born and, to everyone's astonishment and excitement, including Professor Macafee's, she was still alive!'

Needless to say we were all delighted to hear Rhonda's

story. The patient whose bed we were all at just kept knitting throughout my teaching and Rhonda's incredible story, only faltering briefly to smile and nod her head wisely when Rhonda mentioned that her sister was alive and well. Rhonda went on to say that it had been her mother's second labour, and that she had gone on to have another five children, including Rhonda. I suppose you could say that if this baby had been born by Caesarean section, Rhonda would not have been born at all.

Whose baby is it anyway?

Until fairly recently a woman would not have considered herself pregnant until she had missed at least two or three periods, and she would not have confirmed her pregnant state to her family or the world at large until she felt 'quickening', or fetal movements, at around four or five months gestation. Even if she had wished to have scientific confirmation that there was something exciting going on in her womb, she would have had to leave an early-morning urine sample with her doctor, which would then have needed to be sent to a specific laboratory, where the hormones in the sample would have been tested to see if they had the ability to cause ovulation in a small mammal or amphibian. This test could only be performed after three months without periods at the earliest.

Nowadays it is possible for a woman to know that she is pregnant when the fertilised egg has embedded in the uterus, which can be as early as seven days after conception. Whether this can universally be described as true progress is up for debate, but one consequence is that expectations – some would say, unrealistic expectations – of a successful pregnancy are initiated at a much earlier stage. A woman who feels her baby kick definitely knows she has a human life developing in her womb. A woman who sees her baby's heartbeat on the ultrasound screen definitely knows she has a human life growing in her womb. However, when a woman gets a coloured line in a plastic window before or at the time of her first missed period there is a very understandable temptation to hope and believe that all will be well. Expectations multiply exponentially in the days and weeks ahead. Plans are made and often an awful lot of people become involved. Yet upwards of 15 to 20 per cent of early positive results from pregnancy test kits do not develop into healthy pregnancies. I really do believe that we do an injustice to women by not having a health warning on these kits that states in large print: 'There is a probability that there is a healthy pregnancy in your womb. However, it may be some weeks before a viable pregnancy can be confirmed.'

By calling all early biochemical tests 'pregnancy tests', we build up expectations and increase the disappointment and depression associated with loss when it occurs. In the past, a woman told the midwife or doctor that she thought she was pregnant. The doctor would then confirm her suspicion by examination and investigations, and the whole pregnancy was very much a case of a watching brief, hoping that everything would go well, but trying to carefully counsel the potential mother to be prepared if things went wrong.

Nowadays, because of early pregnancy test kits, many women get confirmation that they are pregnant before their body naturally tells them that they are. And when a pregnancy is confirmed, a whole raft of examinations and investigations are instituted, often well before viability has been confirmed. NHS healthcare teams wrap themselves around the woman as soon as the little coloured line shows up. A succession of governments in the last couple of decades has overseen huge changes in attitudes to pregnant women. With expectations of successful outcomes being so high, nature's continual disappointments are now not infrequently turned into legal actions.

We are living in a time of extreme risk aversion and, therefore, almost every action taken by midwives in their statutory role is geared towards identifying problems early and ensuring that the mothers in their charge are as healthy and fit as possible throughout pregnancy. This system works pretty well from a maternal perspective if we regard a successful outcome as being a healthy mother. Personally, I am not so happy with our collective attitudes to the assessment of fetal problems.

Newborn babies die for three reasons: being born too soon, being born with abnormalities or being born too late. The outlook for babies who are premature has improved dramatically in the last decades. In my lifetime the gestation for viability has been pushed back from twenty-eight to twenty-four weeks and the improvement in interventions and attitudes has been both fascinating and a joy to observe.

With regard to the second cause, almost all women are subjected to careful screening to detect fetal abnormalities, and many resources are focussed on those pregnancies to enable the parents to have choices and, where appropriate, to arrange early interventions to improve the outcome for the fetus. This is good not only for the baby, but also for the parents, and for society more generally.

Unfortunately, the area in which we have failed to make much progress in this part of the world is identifying those babies that will die if they are born too late. While we wait for scientists to tell us why all of these babies die, and how to prevent it, or predict that it will happen, one thing we do know is that easily more than 50 per cent of these deaths are associated with poor fetal growth patterns in the uterus. However we are woefully poor at identifying this high-risk fetus in the low-risk mother, to such an extent that among the thirty-three most affluent countries in the developed world, the UK sits well down in the bottom half of the stillbirth league table which is, quite frankly, deplorable.

We don't know why we are so close to the bottom of the table, but we should be trying harder to find out. In Great Britain five in every thousand babies are stillborn; in Finland it is one in every thousand. At a recent national meeting on stillbirth I asked a senior member of the Finnish Department of Health if he could explain the discrepancy, and he replied 'Well, one suggestion could be that in Finland we see the fetus as an individual in its own right, rather than as an appendage to the mother.' Unfortunately there are two obstacles to this approach in the UK. First, there is a widely held belief in the decision-making layer of the health service that a healthy mother equals a healthy baby. To an extent this is true, but current knowledge is increasingly teaching us that late pregnancy fetuses that are stillborn – which are de facto compromised some time before death – are very often found in the wombs of healthy mothers, and their plight is going undetected.

Once doctors and midwives do identify a pregnancy as complicated or 'high risk' we rarely lose the baby. A healthy mother can, however, be falsely reassuring to carers who not unnaturally equate this finding with a 'low-risk' fetus or baby. The big problem is that the method of trying to identify the high-risk baby inside the low-risk mother – armed only with a paper tape measure to determine the size of her bump, and hence apparently the size of her fetus – has been shown to miss over half of these vulnerable babies.

Which brings us neatly to the second problem, which is that some health professionals have perhaps been rather too interested in professional positioning than in the welfare of their charges. When I started in my career, midwives were seen by many as the obstetrician's assistant. In the early 1980s this changed as all concerned realised that the best care a woman and her baby could get was from a multi-professional team of midwives, obstetricians, paediatricians and anaesthetists working together. Antenatal care in particular was almost always a combination of midwives and doctors working together and observing the mother and her baby on a regular basis to the ultimate benefit of all. However, successive policy developments in the Department of Health over recent decades, all directly or indirectly associated with professional positioning under the guise of 'putting mothers at the centre', have resulted in doctors being excluded from apparently low-risk pregnancies, and they now only become involved if and when the midwife deems this could be beneficial. This not only puts a very high burden of responsibility on the midwife, it excludes the doctor from ever meeting mothers who have normal and straightforward pregnancies. How can you detect the abnormal if you don't know what is normal? And vice versa. Forty years on, the obstetrician has become the assistant to the midwife and the role reversal is complete.

This policy is sold to the public as being 'Best for Mothers', when in fact it is actually designed to be 'Best for Midwives'. But is it? Most midwives I know are deeply saddened that they occupy this dominant role and would far rather we all worked together as a team at every level.

My own view is that medics do have a tendency to medicalise too much, and midwives to normalise too much. If medics and midwives are left to work separately from one another, it is the mothers and babies in the middle who will miss out. Working together provides the best of both worlds. Midwives can keep the doctor from being over-zealous in looking for problems, and medics can help improve the identification of the potentially compromised fetus. Both professions can complement each other, as they always did in the past.

Having spent forty years observing the NHS develop I have seen many ideas come and go, and then come back again. I have no doubt that, in time, common sense will prevail, and both the fetus *and* the professions will benefit enormously. Meanwhile we need much more effort expended antenatally to identify the potentially compromised fetus. The advantages of this are immense. If we do identify the compromised fetus before birth, then we can increase non-invasive surveillance by ultrasound and make sure we deliver babies before they die from lack of nutrients and oxygen. Perhaps also we should listen more to our mothers and their concerns during pregnancy.

Joanne, a trusted colleague and midwife gave me an interesting take on antenatal care. She told me the story of Eileen, an ordinary young woman, who found herself to be pregnant. When Eileen was about three months pregnant she happened to meet her friend, a midwife, in the supermarket and told her the good news. Her friend said, 'Have you been to see about getting booked in yet? Have you been taking the folic acid that the government recommends? Have you had your nuchal translucency screen? Have you had your blood tests? Have you had your dietary advice? Hope you've stopped the wine!' and so on. Eileen answered, 'No I have just found out that I'm pregnant and we are delighted with the situation.' The midwife said, 'Oh no, you must go down to your maternity unit and get booked in with your midwife as soon as possible.'

In due course Eileen did go to see her midwife and her GP, both of whom reiterated lots of the advice, and she was given a date on which to attend the hospital. When she went to the hospital she was chastised for arriving late in her pregnancy as she had missed out on the opportunity to have specific tests that were usually carried out at the twelve-week visit, but she did enjoy having a scan, which showed her baby was about fifteen weeks gestation.

She quickly became aware of the large number of incredibly well-versed and well-intentioned health professionals who gave her copious advice both verbally and in the form of endless literature. She was bombarded with information about diet, smoking, drinking alcohol and exercise, all of which was totally irrelevant to her, as she was a fit and healthy woman who never smoked and only had an occasional glass of wine.

She also sat through the parentcraft lessons in which she was told how to travel in a car, how to sleep, what to eat, what to drink, who to attend, and when. Eileen told my colleague that she had found the parentcraft classes a touch patronising, and that the whole concept of the much-vaunted 'choice agenda' relating to childbirth options – regarding pain relief, birth positions and so on – seemed to focus more on the views of the midwife providing the classes than those attending. It wasn't all bad – she 'found the classes helpful, if a bit prescriptive'.

Eileen eventually got to term in her pregnancy. She went into spontaneous labour and came into the local maternity unit where she progressed to a normal delivery of a healthy baby which she breastfed. Initially, breastfeeding didn't work that well, but after the attempts of six different midwives on three different shifts to offer twelve different pieces of advice, (her words, not mine) she managed to get the baby to latch on in a regular fashion.

When the time came to leave hospital, Eileen's husband drove her home. She sat in the back of the car with her newborn baby who was well strapped into a Kitemarked baby seat, having followed the instructions of the absolutely correct health-and-safety-orientated midwife.

At home, Eileen coped very well and enjoyed being with her baby. She was contacted daily by her community midwife, Joanne, who kindly enquired as to the wellbeing of both her and her baby. Ten days after the birth, Joanne called to see her at home and gave her the results of the various tests that had been performed on the baby. Thankfully a clean bill of health was provided and Eileen was very reassured by the news. Joanne checked that her loss from the birth was appropriate, that the breastfeeding was going well and that the baby was growing. The last words that Joanne said to Eileen were, 'Eileen, well done. You have been a model mum and everything has been great. Now don't forget to talk to someone about family planning if you are interested. I look forward to seeing you again'.

Joanne then left, but she was hardly a mile down the road, when she suddenly remembered that she had left some of the tools of her trade, her sphygmomanometer, stethoscope and so on, in the house. She turned the car and went back. When she got to the house, the front door was lying ajar. She went in, and called 'Eileen, Eileen'. When there was no answer, she went in further and pushed open the door of the living room. She was amazed at the sight in front of her.

Eileen had taken all her clothes off, and all her baby's clothes off, and was lying on a big rug in front of a glowing, though appropriately guarded, fire. My midwife colleague said, 'Gosh, Eileen, are you all right?' Eileen just looked up at her and said, 'Joanne, after nine months of state control of my pregnancy, at last I am allowed ownership of my own baby, but I wonder sometimes for how long?'

Eileen just wanted to be alone and do the most natural thing in the world, which is, of course, to be a mother without too much outside influence. While almost all of the care offered (is it really offered, or is it imposed?) to mothers is of true value and very sensible, Eileen's story is a good reminder that the answer to the question, 'Whose baby is it anyway?' is most definitely: *the parents*.

Paddy and Marie

For a woman to give birth to a stillborn child is devastating at any time, but is perhaps especially so when it happens after her due date has passed.

When I set out on my career, ultrasound was in its infancy. Estimating the length of a pregnancy relied on us taking a woman's menstrual and conception history, and on examining her abdomen with our hands. A particularly relevant part of the mother's history, when it came to this estimation, was determining when exactly she first felt the baby move. The first time that a mother feels her baby kicking – that feeling of 'life' or quickening, as we call it – usually occurs at around four months, and is a tangible sign to parents that something really wonderful is happening in the mother's womb. Without exception, every woman I have ever treated was able to give the date, and often the time and place, when she first experienced that feeling. To this day, we are still not sure why women suddenly become aware of the movement of the baby at this particular stage, when the baby has been moving in a similar fashion for many weeks previously.

Working from the date of quickening often proved to be a very accurate way of knowing when the baby was due: simply adding five months to the date provided by the mother was enough to calculate when the baby should arrive. This method has been all but superseded now in much of the developed world by ultrasound. Once the baby's movements do register, the vast majority of mothers will then be aware of movement in their womb in a very regular and increasing fashion. Initially, they describe the feeling as being similar to 'the fluttering of butterfly wings' or, quite simply, 'wind'. Certainly in the last weeks, movement is a regular and constant feature, with many women describing it as possible evidence that the baby is trying to climb out through the umbilicus! So, when a mother reports that her baby is no longer moving, it is of huge significance, and can be the first symptom that the baby's life is over. If that is the case, the mother still has to give birth, but with her expectations, dreams and hopes shattered.

When I worked in the Royal Maternity Hospital in Belfast, a unit which sees 5,500 deliveries per year, around twenty unexpected stillbirths occurred in the final months of pregnancy, on an annual basis. Of course our unit was not unique. Indeed it has recently been calculated that seventeen such babies die every day in the UK. Most of these babies are normally formed and die in the last weeks of pregnancy. At present we often refer to these pregnancies as 'unexplained stillbirths', but increasingly we are finding that there is an explanation, we just hadn't determined it antenatally and therefore did not have the opportunity to intervene. These stillborn babies are mostly undernourished, not because of the poor diet of the mother, but because, for reasons unknown, the placenta has failed to transfer the required nutrients to the baby. Often these babies are a reasonable weight when born, but have failed to reach their growth potential in the womb. One death in particular, that occurred a few years ago, is often in my thoughts.

Marie was eight days past her expected date of confinement. In many countries there is an acceptance that pregnancy shouldn't be allowed to run too long, as we know that the incidence of stillbirth rises quite dramatically when the mother goes more than ten or fourteen days past her expected date. In most institutions, therefore, it is normal to induce labour at around ten days after term. This was what was due to happen with Marie. She was expecting her first baby, had experienced no apparent problems antenatally, and throughout her antenatal notes the midwives had been writing 'fetal movement +, good-sized baby, head engaging' at regular intervals.

However, at the expected date of delivery (term), plus eight days – which was two days before her planned induction of labour – Marie came to the hospital saying that she hadn't felt the baby move since the previous evening. A scan confirmed the worst – there was no heartbeat.

Marie and her husband Paddy were devastated. They came in the next day and labour was induced. Marie was a proud and strong mother and she laboured well, decided against an epidural, and proceeded to a normal delivery of her stillborn baby, a beautiful 3.4kg baby boy, with all the anatomy that should have given him a normal existence.

I had no adequate words of comfort to give Paddy and Marie in those awful days after the delivery, except to reiterate that there was nothing that they had done that could have caused such a tragedy. To carry a moving, growing, beautiful baby for nine months and then have its life taken away leaves the parents grief-stricken, confused, and often understandably angry. We, as the carers, have to search carefully to see if there is something that we could or should have done to prevent these tragedies. Was there some action or inaction that we should have instituted? Were there signs there that could have told us of the clinical tragedy that was unfolding? Often the answer is no.

Some weeks after stillbirth occurs, it is normal practice to sit down with the parents and discuss the pregnancy, antenatal investigations, examinations, and review the autopsy of the baby and the placenta. In due course, I met Marie and Paddy. I remember that Paddy asked the questions, 'Why couldn't Marie have had her labour induced at thirty-nine weeks, when the baby was alive and well? And if she had been delivered then, would the baby be alive and well now?' The answers were pretty simple: there was no obstetrical indication to induce Marie's labour at thirty-nine weeks, and, yes, it was highly likely that had Marie been induced then, their baby would have been born alive.

Paddy's questions were pertinent. Back in the 1970s and 1980s, obstetricians in the UK had studied the timing and causes of all the baby deaths throughout the country, and had been so appalled at the number of stillbirths that occurred in late pregnancy that they wondered how best to address the problem. At about the same time, a fairly new drug, Oxytocin, was introduced into common practice. The drug induced labour contractions when given intravenously (via a drip). Quite simply, the more Oxytocin that was administered, the stronger the womb's contractions. For the first time, obstetricians could accelerate nature! They conjectured that it seemed logical, therefore, that if they induced everybody at thirty-eight and thirty-nine weeks, before they got to the expected date of delivery, stillbirths could be reduced. This system was introduced throughout the UK in the late 1970s and early 1980s, but while it solved some problems it also helped to create new ones. The good news was that many babies, thousands indeed, were born alive that would have died if their mothers had been left to go into spontaneous labour. The downside was that a huge amount of medical intervention was required in order to achieve this outcome.

This medicalisation of childbirth, as many saw it, was very well meant, but was associated with the following problems, which, quite frankly, have coloured my whole time in the profession. First, many women were induced too early or too late because it was difficult to accurately assess gestation. In the 1970s, the estimated gestation of a pregnancy was determined from the date of the start of the mother's last period. This date was notoriously inaccurate as it supposes that all women have a twenty-eight-day cycle and that they all ovulate fourteen days after their period starts, and biology is such that they do not. Also, eggs live a very short time, whereas sperm can be viable for up to a week. A woman could make love hours after ovulation and not become pregnant, yet could become pregnant five days after making love when she ovulated spontaneously. Such is reproductive physiology! Ultrasound was in its infancy, of poor quality, and not available to all. So, instead of inducing labour at thirty-eight or thirty-nine weeks, as was the intention, inevitably some inductions took place much earlier, and others much later. The late ones were not so bad, but the early ones meant that we were creating premature birth problems.

Second, Oxytocin was indeed a wonderful drug that caused uterine contractions, but really, unless the cervix was primed and 'wanted' to be dilated, it was like trying to accelerate a car with the handbrake still on. It produced a lot of noise, but little movement, though eventually the cervix would give in and a vaginal birth would occur. (Thirty years later, we now do have drugs that can let the handbrake off, prostaglandins, but these were not available in 1978.) The consequences were that mothers were in the labour ward for an extremely long time, sometimes days, and so all involved – mums, midwives and the occasional father who braved the surroundings at that time – became mentally and physically exhausted. Caesarean was still a dirty word, as mothers often still had an expectation of having a large family, and so labour was pushed to the limit in order to obtain a 'safer' vaginal birth. Induction rates of 85 per cent during that time were in stark contrast to the Caesarean section rate of less than 10 per cent.

The third problem caused by this new approach was that we now had all the ingredients for an inter-professional disaster. The predominantly female midwives had considered the labour ward as their domain up until this time. They worked well with their male, often domineering, obstetric colleagues, readily summoning them to the labour ward to perform their interventions when they deemed that they were required. But now everything changed. Now male doctors were descending uninvited into the labour ward and taking charge of the mums-to-be, inducing labour, regularly examining them to assess progress and electronically monitoring their fetuses throughout labour.

Many mothers who had yearned for a natural labour were hugely disappointed. Pain relief for mothers was limited almost entirely to nitrous oxide (laughing gas) or injections of morphine-like drugs, as epidurals were scarce. Mothers often had little memory of much of their birthing experience by the time they properly 'came to'. Electronic monitoring of the baby's heart rate had been introduced in the late 1960s and early 1970s and while this was popularised with the best of intentions – to try and reduce the number of babies dying during labour – it was seen by many mothers and midwives as being responsible for a colossal increase in medical interference. And it was. The backlash was mighty and still continues today.

Many of the changes that we have seen in maternity care in the UK have been as a result of this well-intentioned but ultimately unsuccessful initiative in the 1970s. In fairness, the concept of saving thousands of young lives by induction of labour at thirty-eight / thirty-nine weeks was a revolutionary idea and on paper must have seemed incredibly logical. Indeed, for those few years in the 1970s there would have been thousands fewer babies dying after thirty-eight weeks than die today. In retrospect, though, the timing was unfortunate. It was a bit like the cavalry coming through on one day and it then taking about three decades to clean up after it. We are still sweeping up like mad.

Mind you, if we tried the same scheme today, we would have no problems about knowing when a pregnancy was at thirty-nine weeks. We would have no 'jammed-on' handbrakes, thanks to the widespread use of prostaglandins. We would have a population of mums aiming to have one, two or three children at best, and who are not averse to a Caesarean. We would have a population of fathers at the mother's side throughout labour, and we would categorise a labour lasting more than twelve hours as 'prolonged'. Come to think of it, is it time to try it all again?

I gave Paddy and Marie this information to explain why we didn't induce labour at thirty-nine weeks. Then, Paddy said to me, 'Strange you should talk about that, doctor. I was with my mother the other night and she was telling me that when she had me in 1979, she was induced at thirty-nine weeks. She was in labour with me for two days and was pushing for four hours before a doctor delivered me. She begged for a Caesarean section but she said that the doctor told her, "I am not going to perform a Caesarean on you because you are a Catholic, and you will want to have a big family." She didn't agree with the doctor but he proceeded to do a Kjelland's forceps on her, and I was delivered.'

Paddy apparently came out of the birth process in pretty poor condition and required extensive resuscitation. It was only then that I noticed that he had mild left-sided cerebral palsy. His mother was so appalled by the whole birth experience that, rather than risk having a similar experience, she had had no more children at all. Fascinatingly, she had just told Paddy all this as she had wanted to explain to him why he was an only child.

The irony of his mother's story wasn't lost on Paddy and Marie, or on me. If their baby had been born back in 1979 he would have been alive and well because the labour would have been induced at thirty-nine weeks, and well before term +eight days. And if Paddy had been delivered in 2005, he would probably not have cerebral palsy, and his mum would have probably have had two or three siblings for him, because she would have had a Caesarean section for 'poor progress in labour', and would have had a much shorter labour and birthing experience. Much to ponder for all.

The only thing on my mind

There are many areas in my life where I haven't always felt that self confident, but the labour ward was one place where I seemed to develop confidence very early on. From the moment I was granted some responsibility in that environment, I felt comfortable, and enjoyed the challenges presented to me by nature and by my colleagues.

During my training, I was careful not take on challenges that were theoretically outside my remit. However, sometimes needs must. Such a day occurred in June 1976 and the moment has stayed with me because it was, I think, the last time I carried out a fairly high-risk delivery when there was only one thought on my mind. That one thought centred on how I might deliver a baby from a mother safely in such a way that both the mother and baby would suffer no ill effects at all. It was a totally pure clinical goal and it was the only thought on my mind on that day.

I was the senior house officer working at the Royal Maternity Hospital at the time, and it had been a particularly busy day in the labour suite. I had sixteen months experience behind me, and above me on duty were the registrar, the senior registrar and the consultant. The conflict in Northern Ireland was at full tilt, and given that this maternity unit was located in the grounds of the Royal Victoria Hospital at the bottom of Belfast's

Falls Road, not everybody had easy access to our facilities.

On the day in question, three women in the local community found themselves in trouble with their pregnancies at the same time, and three flying squad ambulances had gone out to help, taking with them the consultant, senior registrar and registrar. This left me in the unprecedented position of being the most senior medical person in the unit.

It was about two o'clock in the afternoon when Sister Duffin called me and said, 'Jim, room 4, she is pushing and it's an unexpected breech. First baby.' My heart jumped, and I was quite excited at the prospect of dealing with the situation. I had been taken through the mechanisms of breech delivery by Ken Houston when I was working at the Jubilee unit at City Hospital. I certainly knew what to do, but I hadn't delivered a primigravida breech with no one else around before. I went into room 4 and the mother was doing what mothers do when they have had no epidural and the baby is pressing on their pelvic floor, trying to get out. She was grunting, perspiring and making quite a lot of noise, and all she had to show for it was one very large baby's foot and leg protruding through the birth canal. My first estimate, calculated rather crudely from the size of this one limb, was that the baby looked like it was going to weigh somewhere between nine and ten pounds. I knew that, with the foot and leg down that far, that we had only minutes to make sure that the baby was delivered safely and did not suffer from a lack of oxygen, with all the attendant problems which can emanate from that complication.

There were some brief introductions between myself, the midwife and the mum, and I took over. The paediatrician was called, as was an anaesthetist. Mum's legs were put up into the stirrups and I opened the forceps delivery kit, and then prepared mum, and myself, for the birth. At this point I took a brief pause to go through my mental checklist to make sure that I was ready for any eventuality. I briefly considered whether I was the right person to be doing this procedure, but that particular day I was the only person. I remember thinking of a story that Joe Verzin had told me, about when he was on labour ward in Liverpool for the very first time as a qualified doctor. He too had been challenged to deal with a breech delivery early on during his training, and had got into difficulties delivering the head of the baby. He tried to manoeuvre it this way and that, and initially nothing he tried seemed to work. In desperation he looked up at the sister and said, 'Quick, sister, get a doctor,' to which she replied, 'But you *are* the doctor!' Joe and I both agreed that when you realise this – that you are the baby's only hope – it's incredible how skill, memory, luck, endeavour and perseverance often see you through.

The mother I was now caring for had a partner rather than a husband with her, which was quite unusual as most women we cared for were married, and both of them had realised that things weren't quite going to plan. Very soon after I entered the room, my midwifery colleague and I could see that the baby was a boy. Mum smiled between contractions on being told the news, and dad smiled too! The sex of the baby was of little relevance to the rest of us – we were just thinking that if the baby's head was an equivalent size to its right leg, we could be in for some bother once that part of the baby's anatomy reached the pelvis.

With encouragement all round, mum pushed really well. A second leg was delivered, and bearing in mind everything I had been taught – the most important being 'hands off the breech' – the baby's abdomen and then thorax came into view. I then carried out a Llovsets manoeuvre, and delivered one of the baby's shoulders. Having delivered the baby's anterior (forward) shoulder, I turned the baby around 180 degrees in order to deliver its other shoulder. We now had three quarters of the baby delivered, but we still had what we refer to as the 'after-coming head' to deal with. The trick, I knew, was to let the baby literally hang a while, thus allowing its own weight to gently pull the head fully into mum's pelvis in the correct manner. After what seemed an age, I could see the hairline on the back of the baby's head coming into view. I remembered Mr Houston telling me that this was the time when I was permitted to examine the mother again.

Wrapping a sterile sheet around the baby's torso and legs, I handed the legs up to Sister Duffin, and examined the mother. I can still to this day remember wishing that the baby's head had been a little further down. However, I knew what to do, and although it was the first time I had applied forceps to the 'after-coming head' of a primigravida's baby without anyone better trained at my side, I proceeded to put the forceps on and was delighted when they locked, which meant that the application of the forceps was pretty spot on.

With the help and the continued encouragement of Sister Duffin and the mother's partner, and the huge desire of the mother to get her baby out, along with me putting on a bit of traction, the baby was delivered. A great scream came out from the baby seconds later. Everybody looked at everybody else and we gave a communal sigh of relief and joy. The baby appeared to be as big as I had expected it to be and indeed weighed in at 4.5kg (9lb 12oz) – pretty big for a first baby coming out the wrong way round.

With the baby crying and nuzzling happily in the mother's arms, the happiness in the room, as ever after a good birth, was memorable, heart-warming and a daily bonus that we were blessed to receive. I will never forget the mother's partner, a decent, honest, hardworking Belfast man, who, as he passed me to head off to make the obligatory phone calls, looked me in the eye and gave me a friendly punch on the shoulder and said, 'Thanks, mate, nice bit of work there'. As an obstetrician, the gratitude of happy parents is very hard to beat.

I relate this story because it was the last time in my obstetric career, which went on for another thirty-eight years, when during the delivery the *only* thought in my head was 'I have got to get this baby out intact so it can lead a normal life'. From that point on I became increasingly aware that parents were not going to be happy with just us *doing* our best, but were going to *demand* our best and increasingly attempt to penalise our efforts when we apparently failed to come up to their expectations. Society was changing, and our best efforts were not necessarily going to be good enough for an increasing number in our care.

This approach has, in some ways, been extremely constructive, in that healthcare provision in the NHS is now almost totally based on risk aversion, which has many benefits to it, but at the same time, it has somehow taken out of the arena the purist element of one human being totally and singularly focussed on helping another with no other thought in their mind.

Let me relate an example. Nowadays, in the resourced world – and incredibly in much of the under-resourced world – almost all babies who present breech at the end of pregnancy are delivered by Caesarean section. A huge multi-centre prospective study, coordinated from Toronto some time ago, concluded that, on balance, this was the way to go. Many have been happy to accept that. The skills that many of my generation and before had honed to enable us to perform breech deliveries by the birth canal route have all but gone. Although I am certainly not averse to the liberal use of the Caesarean section, I often wonder whether the scales used to make that decision were calibrated accurately enough before being used. Sometimes, it feels as though the art of obstetrics is being replaced by 'painting by numbers'.

The art, when performed properly, is precisely that – an art form – and I would suggest that most people who choose to venture into obstetrics are excited and eager to perform that art. Medicine and its practice are constantly evolving and I embrace that but I do hope that the craft and skills, and in a way the traditions, of the art are not lost. The common goal of the obstetrician and midwife is to sustain and to give life, so to speak, to the mother and her baby and to do that in the least destructive and most skilled manner possible. The true wonder of birth is ever-present and unceasing and hopefully future obstetricians and midwives will always possess enough flair, craft and art to be equal to it.